Ethics for Everyone

Ethics for Everyone

A Skills-Based Approach

LARRY R. CHURCHILL

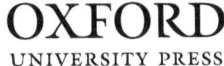

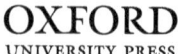

OXFORD
UNIVERSITY PRESS

Oxford University Press is a department of the University of Oxford. It furthers the University's objective of excellence in research, scholarship, and education by publishing worldwide. Oxford is a registered trade mark of Oxford University Press in the UK and certain other countries.

Published in the United States of America by Oxford University Press
198 Madison Avenue, New York, NY 10016, United States of America.

© Oxford University Press 2020

All rights reserved. No part of this publication may be reproduced, stored in a retrieval system, or transmitted, in any form or by any means, without the prior permission in writing of Oxford University Press, or as expressly permitted by law, by license, or under terms agreed with the appropriate reproduction rights organization. Inquiries concerning reproduction outside the scope of the above should be sent to the Rights Department, Oxford University Press, at the address above.

You must not circulate this work in any other form
and you must impose this same condition on any acquirer.

Library of Congress Cataloging-in-Publication Data
Names: Churchill, Larry R., 1945– author.
Title: Ethics for everyone : a skills-based approach / Larry R. Churchill.
Description: New York : Oxford University Press, 2020. |
Includes bibliographical references and index. |
Identifiers: LCCN 2019040688 (print) | LCCN 2019040689 (ebook) |
ISBN 9780190080891 (paperback) | ISBN 9780190080921 (epub) |
ISBN 9780190080914 (updf) | ISBN 9780190080907 (online)
Subjects: LCSH: Ethics.
Classification: LCC BJ1012 .C55 2020 (print) |
LCC BJ1012 (ebook) | DDC 170—dc23
LC record available at https://lccn.loc.gov/2019040688
LC ebook record available at https://lccn.loc.gov/2019040689

This material is not intended to be, and should not be considered, a substitute for medical or other professional advice. Treatment for the conditions described in this material is highly dependent on the individual circumstances. And, while this material is designed to offer accurate information with respect to the subject matter covered and to be current as of the time it was written, research and knowledge about medical and health issues is constantly evolving and dose schedules for medications are being revised continually, with new side effects recognized and accounted for regularly. Readers must therefore always check the product information and clinical procedures with the most up-to-date published product information and data sheets provided by the manufacturers and the most recent codes of conduct and safety regulation. The publisher and the authors make no representations or warranties to readers, express or implied, as to the accuracy or completeness of this material. Without limiting the foregoing, the publisher and the authors make no representations or warranties as to the accuracy or efficacy of the drug dosages mentioned in the material. The authors and the publisher do not accept, and expressly disclaim, any responsibility for any liability, loss, or risk that may be claimed or incurred as a consequence of the use and/ or application of any of the contents of this material

for
David Schenck
ingenious colleague and inspiring friend,
who believed in this book before I did
and
my many students—undergraduate, medical, graduate,
and adult learners,
from whom I have learned so much about ethics

Contents

Acknowledgments	xi
Introduction: Purpose and Uses	1
Why This Book?	1
How to Use This Book: Suggestions for Beginning Students, Professional Students, Clinical Ethicists, and General Readers	4
1. Dimensions of Moral Experience	9
Varieties of Moral Perplexity	9
Curiosity and Wonder as the Impetus for Ethics	10
Ethics Belongs to Everyone	12
The Humanizing Function of Ethical Dialogue	15
Ignorance, Learning (and Relearning) What Moral Values We Hold	18
Ethics as Ongoing	20
Obstacles to Ethics	21
1. Moral Arbitrariness	21
2. Absolute Certainty	23
3. Perfectionism	25
The Aims of Ethics	26
Teaching, Learning, and "Catching" Ethics	28
2. Basic Skills I	31
Probing Skill: Interrogating Our Moral Prehistories	31
Decentering Skill: Taming Moral Vanity and Recognizing Others	38
Relinquishing Skill: Giving Up the Comforts of Moral Certainty	43
Emotional Skill: Learning from Our Feelings	47
Cognitive Skill: Thinking Slowly	50

3. Basic Skills II — 53
   Imaginative Skill: Expanding the Reach of Our Empathy — 53
   Assertive Skill: Claiming Our Own Moral Authority — 56
   Connective Skill: Linking Goodness and Happiness — 59
   Narrative Skill: Story-Making at Intersecting Life Trajectories — 61

4. Exercises Using the Skills — 71
   Nineteen Exercises in Eight Groupings — 71
     Curiosity about One's Moral Sensibility — 72
     Broad Empathy — 73
     Conceptual Agility — 73
     Identifying Emotional Registers — 74
     Sensitivity to Suffering — 75
     Moral Certainty/Uncertainty — 75
     Moral Authority — 76
     Happiness — 77
   Assessing Responses — 77

5. Some Common Pitfalls — 79
   The Trap of Either/Or Thinking — 79
   Expecting Too Much from Theory — 81
   The Desire for a Unifying Definition of Ethics — 86
   Restricting What Experiences Have Ethical Weight — 89
   Treating Mysteries as Moral Problems — 92

6. Moral Concepts in Practice I — 95
   The Anchoring Value of Truth — 96
   Forgiveness and Freedom — 101
   The Varieties of Love — 104
   The Moral Uses of Spirituality — 107
   The Persistence of Hope — 111

7. Moral Concepts in Practice II — 115
   Voluntary and Nonvoluntary Responsibilities — 115
   Justice and the Measure of Impartiality — 118
   Liberty and Its Limits — 122
   Contextualizing Rights — 125
   Conscience: Within—Not Above—the Moral Fray — 128
   How Death Enables Ethics — 132

8. Skills and Concepts for Ethics beyond the Lifespan	137
Skills and Concepts in the Context of Global Warming	138
Five Morally Debilitating Features of Our Current Thinking	141
1. Focus on the Present	142
2. Political Ineptness	143
3. Humans as the Crown of Creation	144
4. Consumerism	145
5. Mechanistic Views of Nature, Including the Human Body	146
Getting Grounded	147
9. Cracking the Case, and Cases to Consider	151
Cracking the Case	151
Cases to Consider (or to Rewrite as Cracked Cases)	159
1. Adderall for Nonprescription Uses	159
2. Programming a Self-Driving Car	160
3. Buying and Selling Organs	161
4. Businesses That Provide Services Selectively	162
5. The Magnifying Effects of Social Media	163
6. Choosing the Sex of One's Children	164
7. Vaccine Refusal: Personal Health and Public Health	165
8. Cows and Global Warming	166
9. Age as a Screen for Expensive Therapies	167
10. Arming Schoolteachers	168
11. Paying Student-Athletes	169
12. Divisive Monuments	170
Notes	171
Bibliography	181
Index	187

Acknowledgments

I am happy to acknowledge, with thanks, the many people who helped in the writing, reviewing, and final production of this book.

This volume has had a long gestation. One of the fortunate things about my entry into ethics is that I was nested in an interdisciplinary department at the University of North Carolina at Chapel Hill. Rubbing shoulders daily with colleagues in the humanities and social sciences, and with practicing physicians, meant that theory could not be privileged in interpreting ethics. My focus necessarily turned to the practicalities of how ethics works and what it means on the ground. I owe much to my astute, early Chapel Hill colleagues, especially to Ruel Tyson, Nancy King, Gail Henderson, Sue Estroff, Barry Saunders, James Bryan, and the late Alan Cross. By the time I arrived at Vanderbilt in 2002, I was firmly entrenched in this more interdisciplinary and useful way to do ethics.

As I began to write in the spring and summer of 2018 I incurred additional debts. Nan and Mark Van Der Puy and Jan Munroe read drafts of chapters and were discerning and encouraging in their suggestions. Keith Meador, Joseph Fanning, and Kate Payne, my former colleagues at the Vanderbilt Center for Biomedical Ethics and Society, offered reassurance that this kind of ethics book was needed. John Churchill, my brother in blood and in philosophy, repeatedly heard many of the ideas in this book over coffee and biscuits. His responses were always thoughtful and heartening. Alan Murphy gave invaluable assistance in refining and sharpening the cases.

David Schenck, my coauthor on several previous books and articles, encouraged me to write about my approach to ethics teaching and learning. His shrewd comments on the initial drafts kept me focused and hopeful that something of value would emerge from what I then called my "quixotic book."

Allison Adams, as with two previous books, was an especially adroit editor. She saved readers from a great deal of academic jargon and challenged me to say things with more clarity. Katie Haywood did extraordinary work in formatting, correcting errant references, and otherwise assuring that the manuscript met high standards for accuracy and consistency.

Lucy Randall, my editor for two previous books with Oxford, had a sure sense for what a book like this might be and how to do it better. I am enormously grateful for her support and guidance. And I owe much to two anonymous readers she selected for reviewing this book. They grasped the aims of the book and offered many suggestions for improvement. I also thank Hannah Doyle at OUP for her diligent attention to detail during the production process.

Much of what I know about ethics I owe to my wife, Sande, and to other members of my family, especially our daughters Shelley and Blair. Over the past decades I have learned from them more than I could have imagined about love, truth, courage, perseverance, joy, and hope. No thanks could be adequate to the deep gratitude I feel toward these three amazing people. I hope they will see some of their influence in the pages that follow. And finally, the emphasis in this book on ethics across the lifespan was inspired by my grandchildren—Miguel, Clara June, Wade, and Sofia. Each has helped me in his or her own way to see how we all change and that our ethical awareness needs to be responsive to these inevitable shifts.

The remaining mistakes and gaffes are entirely my own.

I gratefully acknowledge permissions granted to reproduce small portions of articles already in print.

The section entitled "Conscience: Within—Not Above—the Moral Fray" in chapter 7 is based on my article "Conscience and Moral Tyranny," which was published in *Perspectives in Biology and Medicine* (2015) Vol. 58, No. 4, pp. 526–534. © Johns Hopkins University Press.

The section entitled "Narrative Skill: Story-Making at Intersecting Life Trajectories" in chapter 3 is based on my article "Narrative Awareness in Ethics Consultations: The Ethics Consultant as Story-Maker," *Hastings Center Report* (2014) Vol. 44, Suppl 1, pp. S36–S39. © The Hastings Center. Distributed by Wiley-Blackwell.

Introduction: Purpose and Uses

Why This Book?

This book maps the moral terrain in the grounded reality of human experience without relying on theories or systems of ethics as the primary orienting strategy. Moral awareness needs first to be appreciated for what it is before it is made to conform to theories or systems. And moral consciousness is not a steady or stable set of perceptions; as we change, so do the moral challenges that most concern us.

The point of entry for this volume is the raw materials of moral life—the felt impulses of confusion, perplexity, and moral disorientation, as well as the satisfactions of moral growth and the enjoyments of moral cohesion and consonance with others. This is a book for people seeking to live a life that makes moral sense. It argues that the best way to do this is by practicing and honing certain skills, learning to use some neglected conceptual tools, and avoiding the inevitable pitfalls that oversimplify ethical problems and their resolution.

This is also a book that recognizes that the messy business of trying to live a moral life goes on much longer than most models of ethics typically account for. Indeed, every phase of life seems to present new moral challenges and requires rethinking old assumptions and habits. There are, to be sure, some patches of smooth sailing, but as humans change over time, so do the seas that must be navigated. That means that the exercise of skills for ethics, the meaning of important concepts, and the relevance of various pitfalls are to be learned and then relearned. Their importance must be reassessed at major life junctures.

This way of thinking about ethics as a field of inquiry and activity began for me about 25 years ago when I realized that I was fundamentally engaged in teaching students rather than teaching a subject matter. I was, of course, teaching ethics, as I had always done, but what now motivated me was less a desire to impart the fundamentals of a discipline than an interest in the students themselves, who were often at crucial junctures in their moral development. As I began to play out the implications of this pivot, I became far more interested in what the medical and undergraduate students were saying in class and less inclined to "cover the material." I wanted to hear them out, even when it took discussions in different and unpredictable directions. I became less concerned with whether I had done an adequate job of explaining Kant's categorical imperative and more focused on whether I had met the students where they were, in terms of those moral concerns and interests that emerged in the class. With this focus on students also came less emphasis on reasoning with standard moral concepts and more concern with other skills: how to deal with affective responses to difficult cases, how to accredit and respect—rather than label and dismiss—the differing opinions of others, and generally what counts as growing and maturing morally. The classes themselves became more fluid, less predictable, and thereby more fun, both for the students and for me.

Around that same time, I began anew the practice of clinical ethics consultation in a major tertiary care hospital, following several years of absence from this activity. Listening to patients, families of patients, and those who cared for them professionally was much like listening to students. Both groups—and indeed all of us—enter ethics from distinctive perspectives, with divergent preparations, and with unique histories. The task became respecting and learning from this diversity rather than regulating it into some standard way of proceeding. I also began to see that the key ingredient in "doing" ethics—that is, carrying on the moral inquiry when the class or consultation ended—was curiosity and wonder about one's own moral sensibilities.

With this new approach came the need for different ethics texts, but none satisfied me. Typically, textbooks in ethics written by scholars and teachers of philosophy focus on describing and clarifying the standard ethical theories and rehearsing the customary problem list. In some books, this combination of theories and problems is done with insight and finesse, while in others it seems ham-handed and robotic. But in neither case is it a sound starting place if one wants to make ethics come alive to people where they are, rather than where we want them to be. Such texts usually excel in illuminating only one aspect of moral deliberation: clear-headed reasoning that follows the linear implications of arguments.

One of the things I noted in listening to both students in the classroom and patients and families on the hospital floors is that people are seldom argued out of their moral stances. One reason for this is that moral values reside in places other than our reasoning capacities. They reside as well, and more deeply, in our feelings, our imaginations, and our histories and in the parables, maxims, wisdom sayings, and short stories we tell ourselves about who we are and what we stand for. This book is the result of my search for an approach to ethics in this more multitextured way, a way that will speak to the larger range of human capacities that ethics engages. Ethical reflection is one of the principal ways we become more fully human. This reflection cannot occur if it is confined to reasoning and theory application. We need a view of ethics that engages a broader range of human capacities and one that takes in a wider field of inquiry and activity.

The distinguishing features of this volume are

- a concern with curiosity and wonder as a chief impetus for ethics;

- a focus on the broad range of human moral experiences rather than narrowly on problem-solving;
- ethical activity as requiring a range of skills and capacities and not just clear-headed thinking; and
- an understanding of ethics as changing over one's lifetime, rather than remaining static.

This book is not a guide to problem-solving; it is an invitation to explore the human moral sensibilities. The guidance offered aims at competence in those skills that are necessary for ethical inquiry to succeed. Most works in ethics skip this essential, preliminary step and go straight to a problem list and theoretical applications. Yet if we are to have any appreciation of how theories might be helpful we must first deal with ethics as a complex form of human skills and interactions. This is where ethics begins—and where this volume begins. My goal is to describe some of the basic workings of ethics for the human species and entice readers into an ongoing inquiry into how ethics shapes our lives.

How to Use This Book:
Suggestions for Beginning Students, Professional Students, Clinical Ethicists, and General Readers

Working through the book from beginning to end is one option. Beginning with Chapter 1 can clear away misconceptions and set realistic expectations. I would recommend this approach for first-time ethics students, although other useful strategies for beginners are discussed next. Students with a fair amount of ethics study under their belts will find the skills-based approach of the early chapters adds important tools to their repertoire. Chapter 5 speaks especially to those who tend to get caught up in debates about which ethical theories are best.

Concepts are introduced after the chapters on skills and pitfalls, but you can have recourse to the concepts at any point they are needed. Discovering that you need a conceptual tool to adequately describe a moral experience or analyze a problem is far more effective than being asked to study that concept cold. For example, the first time the term "truth" or "deception" comes up in a discussion is a good time to refer to the section in Chapter 6 entitled "The Anchoring Value of Truth," or when "fairness" emerges in a conversation, the section in Chapter 7 entitled "Justice and the Measure of Impartiality" becomes relevant.

One of the aims of this book is to promote reflection on our own moral experiences and curiosity about the shape and contours of our moral sensibilities. Adult learners typically have many such experiences; students in their late teens have fewer. I encourage readers of all ages to work out of their own life experiences, but this may not always be feasible. One strategy to accommodate for less experience is to go immediately to the 12 cases in Chapter 9 and write a response to one or more of them. Understanding the moral tension in these cases requires no specialized knowledge. This could be followed by working through the first part of Chapter 9, "Cracking the Case," to promote critical reflection on how cases are constructed and how they might be presented from a different vantage point. A second analysis of the cases you select after you have finished the book can solidify and underscore your gains in greater dexterity with moral skills and the ability to interpret concepts.

Another starting point could be the exercises in Chapter 4. Like beginning with cases, this strategy also grounds the study of ethics in something you bring to the course. Efforts to tell a story of how you changed your mind or the difficulties of describing suffering, for example, can then be related to the discussion of the relevant skills in Chapters 2 and 3. Working to get both you and your instructor or conversation partners to invest something that comes out of your lives and experiences is one of the most important features in successfully engaging ethics.

If you are a student in professional education such as medicine, nursing, law, business, or ministry you may come to this book with either a lot of ethics preparation or very little. If you have had a standard ethics course that emphasized the application of theories to vexing dilemmas you will find this skills-based approach more immediately serviceable. Because the practice of your profession routinely requires dexterous personal interactions with your patients, clients, or parishioners, the skills-based approach will find numerous everyday applications. Chapters 6 and 7 can be used selectively. Law students may find the sections on concepts like justice, rights, and responsibilities of greater interest, while students in the health sciences and ministry may find the sections discussing love, hope, and forgiveness carry special relevance.

Clinical ethicists, who do some of the most challenging work I have ever experienced, were never far from my mind as I conceived and wrote this book. In an ethics consultative role, we are almost always constrained by time, by the question or crisis at hand, and by the wide range of patients, families, and health professionals we encounter. For this specialized work the most obviously helpful skills are what I identify as relinquishing, emotional, and cognitive skills, described in Chapter 2 and especially the imaginative and narrative skills discussed in Chapter 3. Finding emotional equilibrium and slowing down the process of ethical deliberation are almost always required in clinical consultative work. Stretching empathic capacities to tell a credible narrative about the issues is critically important. The basic task for the clinical ethicist is modeling these skills and, by so doing, showing that better decisions and better relationships can emerge. Short training sessions can be devised around each of these skills, a task I have begun in the exercises in Chapter 4.

Notwithstanding the professional uses of this text, my aim has been to focus on skills and concepts that are relevant to people not only in their professional roles, but also in the whole of their lives and over the long term. My aim has been to design a book that will not only be worth the initial read, but also worth a second reading 10 years later, as the contours of our lives shift and develop.

1
Dimensions of Moral Experience

Varieties of Moral Perplexity

Life is messy. Situations are sometimes difficult and almost never designed to bring out the best in us. Moral rules for getting us through difficult situations are often too simplistic. Ethical theories that seem elegant on paper often flounder in practice, as though they were intended for robots rather than people. In the lived world, efforts to lead a moral life are beset with perplexities.

"I wish I had done better," we sometimes think. "I could have taken more time, been less emotionally reactive or more patient." Regret over a moral choice is not an everyday experience, but it is common. And beyond larger ethical decisions, the routine tasks of getting around a changing and uncertain world can tax and challenge us morally.

Moral perplexity may take many forms. It may simply be that we wonder why we didn't make different and better choices. We can also be confused about precisely what went wrong or what adjustments would have helped. Or the perplexity may be deeper. Sometimes our actions seem to us (and perhaps to others who know us) uncharacteristic; we may well be wondering what we were thinking. "Was that *me* talking?" we might ask. "It sounded so judgmental." We can also surprise ourselves: "I didn't know I was still angry about that." We can be perplexed about actions taken or not taken, about motives we feel or intentions we have, or about a certain demeanor or stance we adopt. The perplexity can be negative—wondering why we acted so rudely to a friend—or positive, feeling surprised at our forbearance in the face of a belittling remark, or at our courage and perseverance when a family member was in intensive care. Actions and choices get most of the press in ethics, but morality is also about habits, dispositions, and demeanors. Occasionally the demeanors carry a moral message contrary to the acts. For example, cruel actions can be carried out with finesse and aplomb, and kind acts can carry an odor of condescension.

This book is for anyone who has been challenged by these complexities and wondered about the distinctive and fascinating dimension of ourselves we call our "moral life."

Curiosity and Wonder as the Impetus for Ethics

The study of ethics is in large part a response to our natural curiosity about ourselves and fascination with the changing patterns of our lives. Each of us is unique, not simply in terms of an unrepeatable genetic composition, but in terms of our history, our environment, and the influences in our lives. We have a growing sense of this personal uniqueness from an early age, and it is solidified with the recognition that we each are given a distinctive name. Curiosity about just what makes us who we are, the need to explore what is special about us, inevitably involves ethics. Our unique social, environmental, and other influences are reflected in how we size up the world, and ourselves, morally. While our biology may determine much, we are quite open socially, psychologically, and culturally. And our moral norms eventually shape all these ways we remain underdetermined. The desire to explore these unique moral factors that shape us is what drives ethics. In a limited but still substantial sense, we get to choose who we are. Getting serious about ethics begins when curiosity drives us to choose self-consciously rather than by custom or habit. The ethics skills discussed in chapters 2 and 3 can help us realize the potential for choosing a moral life that each of us can call "mine."

Typically books about ethics are packed with problems and the theories calculated to resolve them. Yet most students of ethics do not turn to ethics because their moral systems have run aground by encountering some difficult problem. They turn to ethics because they have encountered others who think differently, or they have a growing sense that they now think differently than they did before college, or before the rotation in the hospital burn unit, or before their much-loved grandmother died. I believe this is also the case for later-life engagement with ethics. For example, living with an intimate partner, or becoming a parent or a grandparent, or retiring, or encountering a serious or chronic illness are all morally charged. In short, whatever life experiences or junctures we encounter carry challenges to our moral sensibilities. While we all face challenging moral dilemmas, the greater impetus for turning to ethics is simple curiosity about these changes and challenges and a desire to understand their significance. When we realize that the moral framework we assumed was stable is actually in flux, we are compelled to study ethics.

A second kind of curiosity and wonderment also motivates ethics: inextricable connections with other people. We are social creatures, intimately associated with others and never free from the need to understand and bespeak who we are, ethically speaking, to family, friends, and even adversaries. To be sure, this sociality can be devoid of wonder if it is imbued with moral arrogance: I assume I am morally superior, so that the views of others do not matter to me. Alternatively, I can block out any real interaction with others if I am obsequious, that is, if my routine demeanor is one of unworthiness, and no praise or positive regard can penetrate my armor of subservience. More productively, this sociality is threaded with a curiosity and wonder at my openness to the ways that others' opinions count for me and help to shape the opinion I have of myself. Am I a *good* son and brother and, later, a good husband and father, a good teacher, scholar, colleague, citizen, and, later still, a good grandfather? Each determination of goodness has its own reference community: the people I look to for insight and discernment. We never cease to be curious about how we are for others and wonder at the intricacies of our connectedness.

A third kind of curiosity and wonderment also motivates ethics. Occasionally we are witnesses to acts of extraordinary moral insight, such as the nonviolent protests for human rights led by Mahatma Gandhi in India and Martin Luther King Jr. in the United States. We not only are deeply curious about and esteem these moral innovations. We also feel a profound sense of wonder and awe at the courage required to enact them. But we need not choose historical or celebrated figures. Most of us have witnessed extraordinary insights and courage in daily matters, such as the challenges of child-rearing, dealing with chronic and debilitating illnesses, sustaining goodwill in the face of degrading attitudes, or perseverance in sustaining care for others that is costly to the caregivers. These insights are also, and equally, objects of our fascination, admiration, awe, and wonderment. And the wonderment isn't confined to acts or people. Reflecting on ethical capacities themselves can bring yet another kind of curiosity and awe. Eighteenth-century philosopher Immanuel Kant said he felt an increasing admiration and reverence for the presence of the moral law within him.[1]

I present this short handbook in that spirit of wonder, fascination, and delight in exploring ourselves as exceedingly complex, dynamic, interconnected, and changing beings. Describing, understanding, and then choosing our defining moral values is the work of each of us and, literally, the work of a lifetime.

Ethics Belongs to Everyone

The ability to act self-consciously based on moral values is one of the defining features of human life. Typically, we learn moral standards from our native environments and our families of origin. As we mature there is both a curiosity and a need to question those origins and decide which are worthy of our embrace, and why. So, while our initial morality from our families of origin is imbibed unself-consciously, at some point morality becomes reflective, and we begin to ask *why* any choice or behavior could be called "right" or "wrong." At this point ethics is about asking and answering, "Why?" What makes a choice or way of life better than the alternatives?

Once the "Why?" question is posed we are off and running, seeking a better, more complete accounting for ourselves than simply saying, "This just seems right to me" or "I have always done it this way." As we grow more comfortable in this inquiring capacity, we learn to ask the question behind that question, and the question behind that one. For example, if I say, "I do it this way because that is what my parents taught me" or "That's what Scripture teaches," I will be led to ask, "How do I know my parents were right?" or "Why should I (or anyone) accept the authority of Scripture?" This does not imply that one's parents or Scripture is wrong. It simply means that ethics probes into why any moral authority should have such influence. Learning to give reasons that, on reflection, are satisfying means learning to think for oneself. At this level, ethics is the desire to know why anything or anyone I accept as a moral authority is worthy of that trust.

Answering the "Why?" question requires stepping back from the immediate context and reflecting, analyzing, probing, and deliberating. And there are many ways of doing this. The idea is to place the problem and the need for an immediate decision "on hold." For example, when we say, "I think I'll sleep on that," we are saying that some gestational time may work well for us, giving us a fresh look at the problem in the morning. In making just this simple move we are implying that the discerning mechanisms we feel are important can be engaged only if we defocus on the immediate and let the problem marinate in our imagination. This simple and typical mode of stepping back lets alternative ways of seeing a problem emerge.

Another way to step back is to consult the authoritative figures in my moral imagination, my moral heroes, and ask, "What would they do in this situation, and why?" I may also gain some critical distance by asking, "How will others look at me if I take one course of action or another?" I can also ask, "Which choices would be worthy of me?" evoking some aspirations I have for my life. Another way of stepping back from the immediate context to find our bearings is to call on the little maxims or sayings that we learned from our moral mentors—often our parents—and see what interpretive sense they can provide us. One of my father's life maxims was, "Do the best you can and take what comes." This epigram encapsulates a combination of a duty to give one's best effort, combined with a stoic recognition that even our best efforts sometimes fail, and we must accept the consequences. It has usually proven to be more useful in my life than standard theoretical analysis. Recourse to parables or short vignettes can also serve the same purpose as pithy maxims or wisdom sayings. One additional strategy most of us use is consulting trusted friends, a dynamic so rich that I will not try to describe it here, except to note that it bespeaks the deeply social nature of ethics, as previously discussed.

Consulting moral theories is yet another way of stepping back and getting some productive distance on a decision. Theories can be very useful for reframing decisions around a feature of ethics, such as happiness or duty, and theories typically provide rules for measuring the extent to which various options satisfy this feature. Theories thus require us to ask, "Which choice will do the least harm and the greatest good, or fulfill my duties in this situation, or which choice is the most just or fair?" Recourse to theories can be helpful, but it is rarely the best way to step back and almost never our first or only reflective move. I will have more to say about the role and place of theories in ethics in chapter 5, "Some Common Pitfalls."

The list of possible distancing moves is very long, and there is no one right way to step back and get this critical distance on oneself and clarify one's ethical priorities. I mention these few to illustrate how to ask and answer the "Why?" question and push ethics into a higher gear. Yet it is important to remember that the space and time for stepping back to reflect is fragile, and it goes against personal habits, institutional inertia, or the sheer need to move ahead and get something done. I will have more to say about this in the section in chapter 2 entitled "Cognitive Skill: Thinking Slowly."

The commonplace moral move of stepping back to gain reflective space carries an important message about expertise in ethics. Ethics is too often thought to be the province of experts—an esoteric field in which the major texts are in Greek or German and in which even the translations are abstruse and the reasoning beyond the ken of ordinary people. I believe there is real benefit to studying great thinkers like Aristotle and Kant, and I devote chapters 6 and 7 to describing some important moral concepts and the innovators who presented them. Yet the lasting insights of these moral theorists can be made accessible to all of us; no advanced degree in ethics is required. More important, the essential practical skills of ethics are already available to most of us and often already in use. The real difficulty is not in understanding them but in practicing them consistently. In sum, whatever the reasons that sound ethical deliberation is so often absent in personal or public life, it is *not* because ethics as a field requires highly specialized knowledge or recondite theories. Ethical reflection and sound deliberation are things that all of us can do, given the will to undertake them.

The Humanizing Function of Ethical Dialogue

An ethical conversation begins with the assumption that others have moral values that are as important to them as mine are to me. I must seriously and respectfully entertain both my conversation partners' values and my own. This simple act is a humanizing activity, for it means that I am willing to set aside, at least for the moment, differences in power, status, and education to consider matters afresh. To be productive, ethical conversations must suspend hierarchy and minimize power differences. Moral values are simply not accessible unless they are approached in this way. This suspension of status to enable attention to values is not easy and is perhaps why genuine ethical conversations between parents and children and between supervisors and employees are infrequent.

Engaging in ethical deliberation means listening—paying attention—and this calls into play our innate empathic capacity. David Hume, Adam Smith, and other philosophers of the eighteenth-century Scottish Enlightenment were the most systematic and sophisticated students of this capacity, which they termed "sympathy" or "fellow feeling."[2] The education and refinement of this universal capacity for sympathy (what we would now term "empathy") through reasoned reflection was for them the core of ethics. Thus, as Hume and Smith saw it, ethics could be said to be humanizing because it called for the higher development of a basic capacity we seem to share with other life forms. Attaining this higher development necessarily requires respectful engagement with other persons as sentient and reflective beings like ourselves whose moral values have for them the same primal place that mine have for me.

Ethical engagement is humanizing in another obvious way. Because it involves the mutual flow of empathy and respectful regard for differences that lets values emerge in an exchange, it is also a mode of interacting that is vastly less harmful to the participants than other modes of handling disagreements, such as shouting matches, holding grudges, filing law suits, or shooting people.

If ethics is considered a mode of conflict resolution, perhaps there is much to learn from studying the moral behavior of other primates. The primatologist Frans de Waal, wary of quasi-Darwinian theories that make aggression the bedrock explanation for primate behavior, has spent a career investigating how relationships are repaired and normalized following outbreaks of aggression. Most rituals for reconciliation, he discovered, take minutes or hours, whereas humans sometimes hold grudges and seek revenge over decades or even across generations. De Waal concludes his book *Peacemaking among Primates* by saying that "forgiveness is not . . . a mysterious and sublime idea that we owe to a few millennia of Judeo-Christianity. . . . The fact that monkeys, apes, and humans all engage in reconciliation behavior means that it is probably over thirty million years old."[3] I will take up the matter of forgiveness again in chapter 6.

The findings of de Waal signal both the immense antiquity of reconciling behaviors and their profound importance for human well-being. Consistent with my previously described approach, it would be accurate to say that while only humans engage in ethics, understood in the deep sense of reflective weighing to guide actions and find justifications, the higher primates are clearly capable of moral activity that is respectful and constructive. I find it helpful to think of ethical discussion and deliberation as a higher form of the conciliatory physical gestures of our primate relatives such as hand-holding, food sharing, and grooming. In other words, our ethical practices are simply a sophisticated verbal and cognitive extension of attitudes of respectful interaction with evolutionary roots extending back several millions of years. Ethics, as twenty-first-century peoples know it, is the most recent flowering of this ancient root.

Moreover, ethical deliberation, as one of the modes of recognition and reconciliation, can have a positive effect on human bonding even when it fails as a mechanism of problem-solving or consensus. Ethics has intrinsic and not just instrumental value, so the benefit of ethical deliberation and discussion can be significant even when consensus is not possible, or an "answer" is not reached. For example, the public policy question of whether to mandate childhood vaccines for attendance at public schools typically places local health officials in opposition to parents who want the final say over their children's lives. While an ethical discussion between health officials and parents may not result in a consensus about mandated vaccines, the discussion can help both sides understand the legitimate concerns of those who disagree. Sometimes a middle-ground position can be found, but at a minimum a mutually respectful attention means that all parties can continue to think of themselves as belonging to the same community.

Ignorance, Learning (and Relearning) What Moral Values We Hold

Ethics is, among other things, a process of learning what moral values we hold. It might be thought that this is self-evident, that we already know what our values are. But the activity of ethics assumes that we do not have such knowledge naturally or that, if we do, we only know in part and that often we are mistaken. Thus, ethics begins with what we might call "Socratic ignorance."[4]

Socrates was the gadfly of ancient Athens who provoked his contemporaries by asking awkward and often unwelcome questions about the taken-for-granted morality of his time. He probed magistrates about the nature of justice, generals about the nature of courage, and the religiously devout about the nature of piety. None of their answers could withstand his scrutiny. And what was true for the ancient Athenians is true for us today. Too few of us have followed our natural curiosity about moral values to explore them thoroughly. Rather, we have settled into some convenient and socially acceptable version of who we are and what ethical standards are worth our allegiance. Socratic ignorance thus expresses the realization that humans generally can be witless about the deeper meaning of the moral values they say they espouse. Socrates thought this was true not just for others, but also for himself. The difference was that he acknowledged his ignorance whereas others presented themselves as confidently knowledgeable.

The Socratic *Dialogues*, written by Socrates' pupil, Plato, detail how such superficial and unexamined claims to knowledge lead to absurd conclusions, personal delusions, and evil. Beginning ethics with an assumption of moral ignorance is important because it leads away from a false sense of moral certainty and toward humility. I will say more about the lure of moral certainty in another chapter, but my emphasis here is upon embracing ignorance because it opens us to curiosity and investigation. The enterprise of ethics is precisely this flow: discovering our ignorance, working through our superficial reassurances of moral knowledge, deliberating with oneself and others on the alternatives for the good life, and finally embracing those moral values which emerge as superior. Socrates is famous for saying that the unexamined life is not worth living, which roughly means that a life shaped by superficial notions of right and wrong lead to delusions about ourselves and others, delusions that are often destructive of human happiness. We will consider later in detail just what sort of happiness follows from living in accord with a search for the best moral values. Suffice it to say that it is not the obsession with materialistic hedonism—bigger houses, faster cars, and higher incomes—of early twenty-first-century Western life, but something more like flourishing, or fulfilling one's best potential.

Our moral sense of self is a large part of what defines us. We hold our moral values, and they in turn hold us. This is not a relationship of reciprocity but of something deeper—an interpenetration. We embrace our moral values, and they leave their mark on us—they enter our thinking and feeling and form habits and patterns that persist over time and, in this way, come to define us. Our "core" moral values, as the name implies, are not external aids, tools, or props we can pick up and then put aside when we are done with them. These central values are simply who we are. Put another way, whatever moral norms we hold position and sustain us in a trajectory, they map us, and following them keeps us "on track." They mark out our path, for good or ill. This is true for both honorable and praiseworthy values, such as generosity, but also for destructive ones, such as envy. Seen is this light, there is hardly anything more important than the kind of probing and examination that ethics endorses.

Ethics as Ongoing

It is sometimes thought that once we have gone through a process of critically examining our moral values we will be set and settled for the duration of life. This would be a safe assumption if we were static creatures. Yet this is far from accurate. Life continues to show that we are moving targets, morally. Changes in our biology, our environment, both physical and social, the structure of our families and our friendships, our professional lives—not to mention all the accidents and unplanned events that occur—all these things change us in multiple and unpredictable ways. And these changes, in turn, affect the moral values we hold and which values we need to adapt, survive, and hopefully flourish. We are simply not the same people we were in a previous period or stage in our lives. Just as no one of us is the same person at 25 that we were at 15, we are different—often dramatically so—at 35, 55, and so on, until our life ends.

Being serious about ethics means being serious about recognizing change in ourselves and others. The virtues and principles of ethics that served us well at one stage in life may not work as well or at all, or may even be counterproductive, at a later stage. For example, the moral values needed for parenting are not the same as those needed for grandparenting. The ethics of being a leader in a business unit are not those of being a novice employee in that unit. The moral values needed for a life in an old age that is diminished physically are not those a healthy 20-year-old needs. This list could be multiplied many times over. The point is emphasized by the pre-Socratic philosopher Heraclitus: change is constant.[5] Adapting the old moral assumptions to the new situation, or perhaps even leaving them behind and discovering new ones, is an ongoing process. Every stage and role in life will bring a new form of moral ignorance, a new need for probing and investigation, and a refined or reworked moral identity.

Obstacles to Ethics

Sometimes moral discussions can fail to launch. These failures are not temporary lapses, such as gaps in our thinking, inattentiveness, or garden-variety pigheadedness, but maneuvers that go off the rails in a wholesale way so that the entire enterprise of ethics is called into question. In various ways these obstacles say that ethics is not just wrong-headed but fruitless and perhaps even impossible. Here are some of the more important moves that barricade ethical progress.

1. Moral Arbitrariness

The idea that morals are arbitrary conventions, or merely custom, is usually labeled "relativism." A moral relativist believes there is no moral truth, just differences. Disagreements between and among people are not grounded in anything real or substantial, but simply reflect social or cultural differences, customs, or perhaps individual tastes. Relativism comes in a variety of forms. A personal relativist might say that what look like moral differences reduce to matters of taste or aesthetics. I like chocolate and you like vanilla. I prefer long hair and wide ties; you prefer crew cuts and narrow ties. In such situations it would be absurd to discuss who is right or wrong. It's just a matter of taste, of what one prefers. Just so in matters of ethics, the relativist argues. There are no common standards we might appeal to, no arguing about moral matters and finding a common resolution based on accepted standards of reasoning. Ethical progress is thus impossible, and ethical discussions, pointless. With personal relativism people can exchange differences of opinion, and this can be interesting, but it doesn't go anywhere.

Social or historical relativists differ only in that they reduce moral differences to cultural divergence and historical contingencies. The cultural relativist might argue, for example, that slavery in the antebellum South was neither right nor wrong, it's just what some southerners believed was right at the time. Saying it was wrong would be an anachronism, imposing our current moral values on a culture that we never experienced. And since relativists don't think moral differences can be adjudicated, they are typically very tolerant of these differences. As Simon Blackburn colorfully puts it, some cultures like to bury their dead, others build little shrines to them, others eat them, and still others worship them.[6] Who's to say who is right about this? It's just different customs, and that's what ethical differences really amount to—nothing more. To be clear, Blackburn has his own arguments against this sort of arbitrariness.

It's important to be able to recognize moral arbitrariness precisely because of its corrosive nature. Claims of arbitrariness make ethical discussion—by which I mean here deliberation and adjudication of moral values—impossible. It reduces ethics to something else, historical or cultural factors, preferences, or aesthetic choices. While stances of arbitrariness may seem cosmopolitan, they often are indicators of intellectual laziness. Intellectual laziness is evident in the resistance to the sort of probing, reflecting, rethinking, and exchanges that real ethics requires. We see people refusing to enter ethical dialogue routinely, sometimes because they have grown cynical but more often because it is just too difficult. I had rather not be asked to rethink my position, thank you very much. The fact made evident by this refusal is salutary, for it reminds us that ethics takes real effort and the exercise of a range of virtues, such as empathy, patience, careful listening, and sound reasoning, as I will discuss later.

Most significant, moral arbitrariness or relativism is a belief system that cannot be adhered to consistently. There are many theoretical relativists but few practitioners. Scratch us deeply enough and on enough topics, and we will always find some matters on which we have strong moral views. For example, students who embrace arbitrariness about sexual matters seem to have a strong sense of fairness and justice about how grades should be assigned. The thoroughgoing relativist, who believes that in all matters ethics reduces to culture history, custom, or preferences, has not entered the ethical dialogue at all, but is taking a metaposition, over and above the fray. To do this completely is to cease to acknowledge what most of us feel is an important part of human discourse. In this sense there are no final, knock-down arguments against relativists, and the best remedy may be to find where their (unacknowledged) moral values are threatened.

2. Absolute Certainty

Absolute certainty can be defined as the direct counterpoint to moral arbitrariness. While the relativist believes there are no disagreements that might be adjudicated by appeal to a commonly recognized standard, those who are absolutely certain believe that there are timeless and universal moral standards that admit to no variation. The relativist believes there is no such thing as moral truths; the absolutist believes there are capital-T truths. While practicing relativists are rare, practicing absolutists are abundant in early twenty-first-century Western societies. An absolutist might believe, for example, that abortions are wrong categorically. They are wrong regardless of circumstance or context, independent of all features that might otherwise mitigate such a judgment. Abortions chosen because of rape, incest, or to spare suffering to a malformed and nonviable fetus are the same, morally, as aborting a healthy, viable fetus for reasons of convenience late in a pregnancy. Absolutists admit no exceptions to the moral truth as they see it.

Moral absolutists are especially susceptible to the notion that following rules is the best way to lead a moral life. "Don't have abortions, or support others in doing so" has the appeal of being clear, easy to follow, and emotionally reassuring. It has the weakness of being too simplistic and failing to distinguish between different reasons and motives for ending a pregnancy. It clumps moral experiences instead of looking carefully at differences between people and their situations. While some moral rules can be useful, moving beyond a moral life that relies primarily on rules to one that is skills-based and encourages skepticism about grand, sweeping generalizations—and the rules that flow from them—is essential if we are to mature morally. We should think of most rules as starting points for reflection, not as commandments for behavior; then we will know which rules to hold on to and which tend to be damaging because they foreclose on thinking and inhibit our growth.

Religious evangelicals and conservative politicians often speak in absolutist tones about abortion and a variety of other issues. Radical left-wing activists often sound just as intransigent. The problem with absolutism as a moral position is that, as in relativism, the enterprise of ethics is rendered useless. An absolutist, knowing the moral truth, sees no need to genuinely engage and turns deliberation, reflection, and debate into castigation of those who differ and conversion to the "right" point of view as the final goal. Why listen to others, weigh their reasoning, or empathize with their perspective if you already know they are wrong? In public settings exchanges with absolutists often begin and end in personal attacks and villainization. This is true across the political and religious spectra; those from the far left as well as those from the far right are both prone to this sort of absolutist self-righteousness. It judges rather than listens; it seeks to convert—to force someone to change their mind—rather than to persuade—to explore other perspectives and possibilities together.

Just like relativism, absolute certainty sucks the dialectical air from the room. It stops conversation and prohibits the emergence of any space for ethical deliberation.

3. Perfectionism

Moral perfectionism is the effort to eliminate all lapses in moral judgments. It is essentially the desire for moral sainthood, for purity. It feeds off a bimodal, all-or-none understanding of ethics. In this way of understanding, "the perfect" is truly the enemy of "the good," or, we might say, "the good enough." In this volume I have emphasized *human* skills, in part to underline the idea that we are morally fragile and limited creatures regarding our ability to live up to our moral standards. Being consistently a good person is an aspiration, not an easy achievement, and mostly we fall short in a variety of ways. Sometimes our moral vision is cloudy; sometimes we use the tools of ethical analysis ineptly; sometimes we are not in command of enough of the facts; at other times we rush our judgments out of impatience or fatigue in dealing with difficulty. Moreover, it is easy to fool ourselves into thinking we are choosing for noble motives, when in fact we are just covering our backsides. The list goes on and on. Ethics relies on a hard-eyed, steady, and candid look at our moral failings, as well as our achievements. Efforts at perfectionism or moral saintliness often turn out not to be noble aspirations, but traps. Since perfection and saintliness are impossible they often lead to cynicism, as our superhuman standards result in constant failure. A moral standard impossible to meet will be eventually discarded.[7]

Yet there is another conclusion even more disturbing. Saintly aspirations can also lead to moral self-delusion—thinking we are better than our actions warrant. Perfectionist aspirations in medicine, for example, make us less aware of the ways claims of altruism in patient care cloak self-interest. The same might be said for parenting. Montaigne had a pungent way of expressing this: "There are two things that I have always observed to be in singular accord: supercelestial thoughts and subterranean conduct."[8]

Perfectionism as a way of thinking about ethics can apply to communities as well as individuals. Western political thought is replete with visions of perfect societies, or utopias, and they stretch from Plato's *Republic* to Karl Marx's vision of communism. Thomas Nagel has rightly critiqued this form of collective perfectionism: "A theory is utopian in the pejorative sense if it describes a form of collective life that humans, or most humans, could not lead and could not come to be able to lead through any feasible process of social and mental development."[9] Thus does utopianism engender impossible perfectionist tendencies. It always flounders because of the complexities and fragilities of human life.

The Aims of Ethics

Ethics has four aims. First, it is a way to discover and rediscover our own values, then to choose them, and finally to live by them. Ethics results in knowing what we value and why we value it. Second, ethics aims to discover the moral values of others. We are led to this discovery because understanding the moral values of others is part of the process of uncovering our own. I cannot simply reflect on my moral values and then identify them through introspection alone. The French philosopher René Descartes thought he could go into social isolation and identify the roots and warrants for true knowledge.[10] The results were disastrous. Going into hibernation to discover my moral values is equally fruitless and hazardous, leading to a dehumanized model for knowledge. In ethics we need conversation partners; we need the company of friends, spouses, children, and neighbors and a wide range of thinkers, poets, and literary texts to even sense the possibilities of what moral values we might entertain as fitting for ourselves. Thinking deeply means having thought from the point of view of others, far and near, living and dead. Ethics thus aims for understanding others' moral values both as instrumental to getting my own head clear and as an end in itself.

A third aim is to achieve accord between our internal moral lives and our external actions. Behaviors and choices rarely reflect the full moral weight we assign to them, or all we intend them to convey. Hence, the constant need to say what we intended, wanted to achieve, or were trying to do: "I only meant to help," we often say when our well-intended actions make matters worse. Or, "I am doing this for your own good," we say when we need to justify usurping someone's prerogatives for an end we somehow "know" to be better than what they would otherwise have chosen. Praiseworthiness and blameworthiness of actions often depend on how they can be interpreted through recourse to some feature of the inner life we want to make visible. Ethics then aims for clarity about the nest of motivations and intentions that accompany all moral behaviors, about the complex gestures—both verbal and bodily—we employ to make ourselves transparent, both to others and to ourselves. Consonance between our inner moral sensibilities and our exterior actions puts us at rest.

Finally, and most obviously, ethics aims to solve problems. Problem-solving is sometimes thought of as the most important, or sole, aim of ethics. I have placed it last to suggest that it may well be less important than the other previously discussed aims. Certainly, if the other three aims are achieved, problem-solving becomes less problematic. Sometimes we don't so much make a decision but realize that in the process of achieving the first three aims of ethics, a solution has been reached. Problem-solving is then more like a discovery than a decision.

Teaching, Learning, and "Catching" Ethics

Skepticism about ethics abounds. Everyone who takes ethics seriously will at some time encounter people—students, colleagues, friends, administrators—who are skeptical or even dismissive about the whole enterprise of ethics. For example, medical school curriculum committees on which I have served occasionally embraced a false dichotomy between the "hard sciences"—physiology, biology, chemistry—and the "softer" subjects covered in the social sciences and humanities. The idea is that there is real knowledge in the former disciplines and only conjecture and opinion in the latter ones. Too often this caricature of disciplines and dismissal of ethics is accompanied by a model of intellectual and social maturation that overemphasizes the developmental tasks of adolescence and ignores everything that follows. The notion that "these kids have their ethics when they arrive. Not much we can do to change them at this late stage" captures this psychological paradigm and the moral determinism that follows in its wake. Thus conceived, the aim of medical education becomes one of admitting "good" people and filling them with the knowledge base of scientific doctoring. And a similar case is sometimes made for other professions, such as law, nursing, engineering, and business. Such a belief not only is overly simplistic but endorses impoverished moral norms embedded in this industrial view of education. Most people with whom I have worked do not see themselves as morally finished products, needing only the addition of technical knowledge. Nor do they see ethics as intended only for the soft-minded. My hope is that the concepts and skills of ethics described here will nurture both a conviction of the importance of ethics and a sense of being ethically unfinished and thereby make us more open to new learning.

Finally, one occasionally hears, usually in turgid tones, the view that while ethics cannot be taught, it can be "caught." That is, personal and professional mentors can model good behavior, and in that way we learn ethics by imitating our wise masters. This view has always seemed to me a little self-congratulatory. Mentors vary widely in their professional and personal virtues, and there is little assurance that growing and developing persons—in the absence of the critical reasoning tools of ethics—will copy a virtuous and thoughtful person rather than a clever and self-serving moral imposter. Even the field of ethics itself shows the hazards of assuming students will "catch" ethics. Ethics professors with notorious personal standards are not hard to find. Catching ethics is possible but only when one is selective about the source and encouraged to get critical distance on the behaviors being modeled.

2
Basic Skills I

There are no child prodigies in ethics. Experience is required, along with facility in a diverse set of skills. Listed in the following discussion are some of the fundamental practical skills we need in ethics. These capacities enable us to use moral concepts and principles with greater ease in problem-solving and, more generally, in orienting us morally. Like cooking, carpentry, tennis, or poker, these are skills that can be learned, practiced, and refined. Most skills require years of practice to master. Ethical capacities are no different. They require learning and relearning over the inevitable changes of the lifespan.

This skill list can be considered a response to the question, "Why do ethical discussions so often go into the ditch and become unproductive and frustrating?" One answer is because those engaging in moral deliberations fail in the exercise of one or more of the capacities listed in the following text. Without these skills, ethical reflection never gets very far.

These skills are named according to the capacity they engage in us: *probing, decentering, relinquishing, emotional, cognitive, imaginative, assertive, connective,* and *narrative*. This is a basic list, not an exhaustive one. I hope readers will refine this inventory and enumerate other important skills I have neglected.

Probing Skill: Interrogating Our Moral Prehistories

"But Prof. Churchill, you're asking me to question my faith in God, and I don't want to do that."

Some remarks from students reverberate in my mind for years. Resistance to critical thinking is not unusual, but rarely is it vocalized with this kind of candor. Yet coming to any degree of ethical maturity means being willing to overcome this resistance and investigating the assumptions of the moral frameworks each of us has inherited from our families of origin. These frameworks constitute the moral dispositions and beliefs that are simply taken for granted and often function unwittingly as the "good" or "right" way to do things. Of course, for some people, the act of probing itself is forbidden and is tantamount to the rejection of the moral standards embraced in our families of origin that have made us who we currently are. This taboo makes the study of ethics difficult, if not impossible. Likewise, if my current, individual moral identity has been forged in a hard-fought rejection of the standards of my parents and the nested moral assumptions that permeated my youth, I may be very protective of this new identity and loath to examine it. In this latter case, teachers of ethics can be mistaken as parental figures, championing the old morality, rather than probing for what makes any morality worth our devotion. This is all to say that wherever we begin the serious study of ethics, wherever we are on the road to learning to think for ourselves, the challenge is the same: achieving enough critical distance to investigate one's own moral sensibility, describe its framework, and probe its workings. The task is always to discern what we think and believe and then see if it will stand up under scrutiny. This is what ethics is all about.

We all enter the study of ethics with a wide range of predispositions and beliefs. Some of us are devout Catholics or Baptists, and our ethics is essentially what we understand the teachings of these traditions to be. Some of us have rejected those belief systems and their accompanying moral teaching. Some of us grew up in households and social environments in which religion was thought to be unimportant for ethics. When this is the case, we may think of ourselves as reasonable, considerate people living in a pluralistic world in which tolerance of differences is the cardinal virtue. Some of us early became disciples of Ayn Rand or Milton Friedman; some of us are casual hedonists, seeking to find our pleasures without bothering anyone else too much. Many of us hold residual racist or sexist views (*residual* because we have made some efforts to recognize and free ourselves from racism and sexism); some of us view the world with moral suspicion; others, with a demeanor of trusting acceptance. By late adolescence many of us harbor some degree of anxiety, perhaps even guilt, simply because we no longer live by some of the standards we were taught in our childhood and are tacitly seeking absolution, or perhaps justification, for the breaks we have already made from our families of origin. Some of us are unvarnished idealists, hoping to find a way to make the world better, but we are yet unprepared for the ways our ideals will be tested or compromised by the bumps and bruises of living. And to varying degrees and in diverse ways all of us occasionally resist probing into our moral predispositions, as did my previously quoted 18-year-old student.

This is just a small sampling. My point is that entering a study of ethics means—at an absolute minimum—taking the initial step of embracing a critical interrogation of some of the assumptions about right and wrong, good and bad, with which we begin. And it isn't just a matter of which moral values are held, but also of *how* they are held—tightly or loosely, with conviction or casually, close to our hearts or largely in our heads. How to initiate and sustain such an inquiry—an inquiry robust enough to make us both curious about and critical of our moral predispositions—is the art of ethics. And it must never be forgotten that the eventual task is to make each of us able to go on, doing the critical thinking of ethics, after the initial probing has ended.

There are many moral development schemes to choose from, but few of them address the most crucial step in ethics,[1] which is interrogating one's moral predispositions, what I will term here as one's "prehistory."[2] We each carry our moral prehistory like a backpack: It contains valuable things, but it is mostly out of sight. One important feature of the prehistory backpack is that it has been stocked by someone else, usually one's parents, but also by grandparents, aunts and uncles, cousins and friends, schools, and social and religious organizations—really, many influences and in a differing mix for each of us.

The contents of the backpack may be not only conceptual but also physical and topographical. Physical places often seem to exude their own moral meaning, so that "getting grounded" ethically has both metaphorical and literal meanings. It is no accident that moral changes often follow not only bodily changes—such as those that accompany physical maturation, growing older, or becoming less able—but also moves in location from one home to another or one region of the country to another. The writings of Wendell Berry about Henry County, Kentucky, are vivid illustrations of the way moral epistemologies are embedded in the local soil or reside in a landscape.[3] This point is made elegantly in Keith Basso's study of the Western Apache: "Wisdom sits in places."[4] Moral landscapes can be both interior and exterior, both figurative and literal. The ways both our moral imaginations and our early behavioral habits are configured by and interact with the physical topography of our place of origin may well be an important component of our moral backpacks.

What we all have in common is that we didn't get to choose the contents of our moral backpacks ourselves. They were loaded for us before we had an identity solid or clear enough to know how to choose. Indeed, even though the contents may be a haphazard, jumbled accumulation, in large part this moral backpack gives us enough initial self-identity to even know that choosing is possible. Hence, the moral backpack belongs not to our history but to our *pre*history, and there is little motivation to swing it around, zip it open, and make it the focus of our gaze until we encounter its limits or inadequacies. As we grow, the moral backpack can seem too light, without the requisite moral tools for living a full life, or too heavy, with excessive, burdensome, or even toxic contents—or both.

Recognizing the possible limitations of my own prehistory is the first and most necessary movement in the human enterprise of ethics. In some ways this movement is the most difficult, for it means breaking the shell of moral naiveté. It can be as simple as seeing for the first time that one's friends were reared in households with different life priorities, but it continues in a range of recognitions. For medical students, it may be an encounter with their first hateful, angry, or drug-seeking patient, or the recognition of how little influence they have over the health of many of their patients. In child-rearing, it can be an abrupt realization that my spouse or partner and I have unself-consciously imbibed very different understandings of what children need and how to instruct or discipline them. Everyone has their own personal list of these pivotal events. We should honor and prize these often-difficult realizations, because without them we never learn to think for ourselves; without them we never learn the sound of our own moral voices, rather than all the others in our heads vying for the place of moral primacy.

A caveat to forestall misunderstanding: interpreting this most basic move in ethics as one of learning to think for oneself may seem to endorse a detached and solitary individualism as the end point of this shift toward maturation. While this movement is part of what stamps us as distinct individuals, it does not lead to the kind of individualism that stands over and against communal life. Breaks from communities of origin are almost never complete or total. This dynamic is in fact best described not as a break but a pivot, a shift in perspective that permits an assessment of moral prehistories, and a fresh and more clear-eyed engagement. Inevitably, this assessment will also mean a shift to a somewhat different community of moral reference. Moral selfhood is not just accidently, occasionally, or contractually social but fundamentally and irreducibly social.[5] A typical part of this initial displacement is some degree of *re*placement into the community of moral origins, now seen with new eyes, but also engagement with other communities from which I can draw an enlarged sense of self and an expanded notion of ethics.

My assumption is that one is never really finished with this examination, shuffling, and repacking. Each age in life seems to bring new problems, or at least questions not evident or considered important in earlier times. As a result, we encounter new points of entry into the inherited moral sensibility and thus more opportunities to learn new processes and skills for meeting these new challenges, entailing altered priorities and a novel form of homeostasis. As life moves on we may come to recognize these homeostatic points as temporary. Life does not stop, and neither does ethical discernment.

I also assume in this description that no backpack is ever fully emptied and examined. Some elements simply lie too deep within our moral sensibilities and thus are opaque to our most rigorous efforts. Despite the high optimism of some philosophical traditions, it seems clear that humans have no transparent window into all the features of our personal moral scaffolding. But the practical incompleteness of moral self-scrutiny doesn't mean that all effort at moral self-awareness is futile. For most of us, the moral life is marked by recognizable transitions, both large and small. The key issue for ethics is resistance or engagement. Resistance usually leads to moral stagnation; engagement is typically the first step of growth.

In brief, if there is no questioning, no probing of prehistory, no curiosity about the adequacy of what one has inherited morally, then we never have the occasion to rethink and thus grow morally. Moral problems will be either largely denied, or those with different views will be judged to be wrong. The 2016 presidential election and the politics surrounding it are sad confirmation of how difficult and personally threatening it can be to seriously entertain views that differ from one's own. But the price for hiding within one's moral shell is a high one. The cost is moral isolation—withdrawal from moral dialogue and a fortified moral insularity. Religious and political enclaves are prime examples of this strategy, in which rethinking is a sign of unfaithfulness and disloyalty, and any questioning of the moral authorities of the group leads to expulsion from the community. Those who dare to breach the echo chamber are labeled "not genuine Christians," "not true Republicans or Democrats," or "not real Americans."

The student quote that opens this section may have been voiced out of such a tribal fear. I do not know. I do know that her religious faith provided such a powerful security that when I asked the reason for her confidence that religion had provided all the moral answers, she thought I was requiring her to question her faith. And because her faith was so tightly held, questioning it was for her the same as rejecting it. Her response shows us what we lose if we never interrogate our moral prehistory. It forecloses the metalevel engagement of morality, the entry into ethics proper, understood as the ability to step back and ask questions about our native moral orientation. Without the willingness to undertake this critical reflection, we are confined to our inherited moral intuitions. Ironically, unless we can interrogate our native moral sensibilities we will never be able to recognize their value and authentically embrace those features of it that can withstand scrutiny. Ethics is never just what we do; it is also understanding *why* we do what we do.

Opening the moral backpack to critical scrutiny is not without risks. Studying ethics is best undertaken when our conversation partners are curious and welcoming and the space of inquiry safe enough for us to do some unpacking. The environment and one's fellow inquirers must also be sufficiently open to differences so that new insights may emerge and be taken seriously rather than summarily dismissed. Public conversation in the United States seems to have less and less space for this kind of honest rethinking and nonjudgmental disagreement.

In brief, breaking the shell of moral naiveté is essential to moral growth. It puts us in a different place; it broadens our moral horizons, bringing into view a larger world and, at least potentially, an enlarged domain of "right" and "good."

Decentering Skill: Taming Moral Vanity and Recognizing Others

When we interrogate our moral prehistories, a second skill comes naturally into play: curbing and calming our moral vanity. Most of us not only have a good opinion of ourselves morally, but we also have a major investment in the belief that we are good people. We often fall prey to a distorted self-image. As David Brooks says, we "grade [ourselves] on a forgiving curve."[6] The need to think of oneself as genuinely good, sometimes despite lapses and appearances to the contrary, may in fact be an early moral teaching perpetuated in adult life. In the face of clear wrongdoing, many of us as children were told that the deed was "not worthy of us," that we were acting "out of character," that we are "better than that," and so on. These are all variations on the effort to separate an essentially good self from the bad action and thus shield our core moral identity. Even in adult life we are usually hesitant to call someone evil, and we speak instead of the actions, attitudes, behaviors, or choices, rather than the person, as morally deficient. This hesitance is simply part of foregoing judgment about the deep inner moral core we want to protect in both ourselves and others. And this is certainly a useful strategy, but it can be taken too far. In its toxic form, this separation of action and attitudes from a protected core self is an exercise in vanity and a denial of responsibility.

Consider, for example, occasions in which we attribute questionable motives to others but not to ourselves for the same actions. One instance of this double standard is the findings regarding physicians' perceptions of the influence of accepting gifts from pharmaceutical firms. Surveys have consistently shown two things. The first is that physicians generally consider themselves immune to the influence of gifts that are small in value, such as pens, notepads, meals, or small favors for clinical staff. A typical response to the idea that a meal paid for by a drug rep could influence prescribing behavior is, "I can't be bought for a pizza."[7] The American Medical Association

(AMA) guidelines for physicians on accepting pharmaceutical gifts suggest that those of small monetary worth are not ethically problematic.[8] This guideline reinforces a general consumerist valuing of gifts based solely on price, as if the relational and bonding power of giving and receiving doesn't matter. Studies have shown, however, that no gift is too small to have an impact.[9] Equally important, the tone of the AMA's recommendation legitimates a common feeling among physicians that they are such high-minded people as to be above all that. Lois Shepherd presents a convincing argument that in fact the touted altruism of doctors may serve as a moral blind spot of exactly the sort I am addressing here.[10] If both the public and doctors themselves assume that physicians operate out of altruism to an unusual extent, then self-serving actions are less likely to be interrogated. Moreover, they are more likely to be miscategorized as altruistic, when in fact they are simply self-interested. The second finding from physician attitudes about pharmaceutical gifts indicates even more clearly the toxic effects of moral vanity. In a major survey, many physicians said they were worried that their colleagues might well be inappropriately influenced by such gifts, but that they themselves were not.[11]

Overestimating the benevolent aspects of our motivational complex is, I believe, a general hazard and perhaps a special hazard for those whose social role and professional self-definition routinely calls for altruism.

I do not argue that all high moral self-regard is necessarily bad and certainly not that a solid moral self-respect is problematic. I do not argue that vanity must be rooted out, but rather that it must be tamed. And taming it requires a process of decentering—dislodging ourselves sufficiently from our self-love so that we can distinguish the useful from the toxic. A certain good opinion of oneself is likely an enabling element to make it through the tough patches and to recover after moral lapses, from which we all suffer. Yet, as Simon Blackburn argues, an excess of vanity makes us even more vulnerable than we already are to the commercial enticements that routinely prey upon our self-love.[12] This vulnerability to consumer blandishments might be reason enough to reconsider the extent of our self-affection. My focus here, however, is on the ways excessive vanity always involves self-deception. More precisely, I am concerned with the moral impact of that self-deception, in the same way that narcissism is antithetical to accurate moral self-awareness.

In Greek mythology, Narcissus is drawn by Nemesis to a pool, where he falls in love with his own reflected self-image. Taking this reflection for reality, Narcissus is thereby doomed to unwitting and unrequited self-love—and by implication a truncated capacity for engaging both self and others appropriately. Among other things, narcissism places severe limits on empathy. Narcissus chased his fantasy lover relentlessly, and in the end, he drowned in pursuit of it. Thus does the vanity of narcissism come to a dead end—a full stop for any movement toward ethical awareness and maturity. Empathy, the skill of imaginatively entering another's thoughts and feelings, clearly depends on displacing oneself from this terminal version of vanity.[13] Taming our moral vanity means seeking communication with and care for concrete others who are not simply mirror images of oneself.

Skills of decentering refer to more than a basic realization that my words and actions may affect others, for good and for ill. Imagine that we jointly agree to share a set of garden tools so that neither of us will have to purchase the spades, picks, pruning shears, and other instruments needed for each of us to maintain our gardens. If I leave the shears and shovels out in the rain rather than storing them properly, I have failed to live up to our agreements, damaged the tools specified for common use, and perhaps jeopardized our relationship as well. But this is not the same as recognizing you as a moral agent like myself. So far, this is just recognizing that my actions can affect you, for good or ill.

To recognize you, in the full sense of seeing and understanding, as a moral agent means that I understand that you, like me, are a center of consciousness, with a history, values, life priorities, wants, fears, aspirations, and goals, indeed with the entire panoply of human attributes that I find in myself. When I begin to see you as a moral agent, you are morally alive to me, complex rather than simple, and I discern that you are as alive to yourself as I am to myself. In this sense of being-alive-as-embodied-moral-selves, we are equals, individuals on the same plane of life.

Returning to the example of the shared garden tools, when I see you as a vibrant and complex person—much like myself—I understand why your anger toward me for neglecting the tools is justified. I have mistreated not just the tools, but you. You wonder if I can be trusted. And repairing the damage will mean that I not only replace the damaged tools and pledge to do better in the future but make good on this promise. A tool-sharing relationship is a microcosm of the thousands of interactions in which the full and mutual moral presence of both people is needed.

Around the hub of this recognition of other people as moral agents, one can gather a large range of strategies for relating to others—ways that seek to honor their selfhood, to let them know, in ways obvious and subtle, that I see something of who they are. I respect them, as I hope to be respected. Around this basic insight can be gathered norms of respect, tolerance, reciprocity, cooperative strategies for fairness and justice, and a host of others.

Too elementary, you might be saying. Everybody knows this. But I very much doubt that everyone does know this, or at least know it well enough to avoid using others for one's own purposes, regardless of the harm or disrespect that others may feel. Elected leaders, both local and national, routinely act as if some others do not count, and they treat some groups as something less than full centers of moral consciousness and thereby equal—in this way, if in no other—to everyone else. In *Democratic Vistas*, Walt Whitman, writing in the aftermath of the American Civil War, saw clearly that the failure to recognize the moral agency of others was destructive not only of ethics but of democracy: "Of all dangers to a nation . . . there can be no greater one than having certain portions of the people set off from the rest by a line drawn—they not privileged as others, but degraded, humiliated, made of no account."[14]

To see others as moral agents is to see that I am not the moral center of the universe. I count, but others count as well, and in collective and social situations (in contrast to my private life), we all count equally. It is this insight that John Stuart Mill had in mind when he insisted that in the utilitarian calculus for happiness, each counts as one and no one counts as more than one.[15] There is something of this in Kant as well. He insisted that we act on principles that we think should apply to everyone; don't make exceptions for yourself. This is the meaning of universalizability.[16] For Kant, asking, "Should I do it?" requires also asking, "Can I will that everybody do it?" Ethics is the ongoing effort to unprivilege myself.

The recognition of others as full moral selves leads naturally to the question of who is included in the designation of "other." Others who look and act like me? Those like me in socioeconomic status, age, race, gender, or, increasingly, those like me in political persuasion? When Mill was writing, it was assumed that the important others to whom I would grant full moral agency were male and very likely landowners. Slavery ended in most of the British Empire in 1833, but the British Parliament didn't pass an act granting women the right to vote until 1918, and even then, there was a social status restriction. Women granted suffrage were those over the age of 30 who were householders, the wives of householders, occupiers of property with an annual rent of £5, and graduates of British universities. It took more than 30 years longer for slavery to end in the United States, following the bloodiest war in American history. American women were enfranchised to vote after the ratification of the Nineteenth Amendment to the Constitution in 1920. The struggle for full recognition of women in society continues as I write. Equal pay for equal work is still not realized, despite the work of people like former U.S. presidents Carter and Obama and Supreme Court Justice Ruth Bader Ginsburg.

These short histories are important to illustrate two things. One is just how recent the gains in basic human rights are. Another is how grudgingly these rights have been granted. Preceding each legal enfranchisement was a moral recognition that at least some "others" (African Americans and women) were sufficiently like the ruling class that they deserved inclusion. Full moral recognition of the kind I previously discuss is still not a part of the social fabric for many, as residual (and sometimes blatant) racism and sexism still exist in parts of both the United Kingdom and the United States. The Montgomery, Alabama, memorial of racial terrorism is a sobering reminder that even after slavery ended in the United States, atrocities against black men were customary. Over 4,000 African American males were lynched between 1877 and 1950, for "offenses" as trivial as using the wrong tone of voice when addressing whites.[17] The full recognition of the moral agency of others is a slower process than what can be accomplished by changes in laws, desirable as these legal changes may be.

The moral decentering of the self is inevitably followed by some sense of reorientation, gaining one's moral bearings in a community that now includes others. One measure of moral progress is how we answer the question, "Who, among the others, do we include in the circle? Who are members of the community that we recognize as moral equals?"

Relinquishing Skill: Giving Up the Comforts of Moral Certainty

In the opening chapter I discuss "absolute certainty" as an obstacle to ethics. There the argument is that such certainty brings the conversation to a halt. Here I discuss a less absolute form of certainty, but one that still harbors dangers for the work of ethics. The skill involved here I have labeled relinquishing or surrendering that sense of deep satisfaction, even pride, that accompanies the conviction that we have done the right thing. This is not an argument against seeking moral certainty. It is an argument against the comfort that follows from believing we have arrived, precisely because that comfort will prohibit us from probing further. Ethical deliberation, of course, always must find a resting point; otherwise, we would never act and would be caught in endless cycles of deliberation and rethinking. Yet the resting point, even when it eventuates in decision and action, should very rarely have the stamp of finality. As one of my early career mentors, Harmon L. Smith, put it, "In ethics we need the courage to be decisive without the pretense of being definitive."

We have all experienced the gratification of thinking we were right—that deep certitude that among all the tempting lesser choices we might have made, we chose the right path. But herein lies a substantial hazard. Just when we want to rest on our laurels, we should be probing for ways we may have been lulled into moral complacence. One helpful maxim is this: "Be most suspicious when you are the most certain." This is not to dispute the fact that people sometimes believe they are right—and indeed, on closer examination, they *are* right. They have done their empathic homework; they have worried about prejudice, narrowness of values, misunderstandings, lapses in reasoning, and emotional philistinism, and, sure enough, they have made a judgment they can admire. My worry is not about this phenomenon, rare as it is, but with the desire to skip steps—to feel this assurance and the moral comforts it affords without the hard work it takes to get there.

Certainty is often the result of oversimplification of the issues, moral sloganeering, and reliance on a few pet principles, rules, or maxims to the detriment of a full, deliberative process. The culture encourages us to do precisely this sort of ethical short-circuiting. We are daily offered moral issues in black and white, devoid of nuance or circumstance. For example, we are encouraged by many to say that all abortions are wrong, that all taxes are bad, that freedom of choice is an unqualified good, and so forth. The list is very long. Even the best reporting in news programs is frequently framed in precisely these terms, with two opposing experts espousing predictable and simplified positions.

In a recent essay assignment, I asked a group of honors college undergraduates to write on the seven most important moral concepts for understanding the abortion debate in modern American society. Part of the task was to list these concepts in order of their priority or, alternatively, to draw a diagram of how these seven terms are interrelated and explain why a serially ordered list of concepts will not work. Most students found this difficult, but all found it illuminating. They were forced to think outside of the "either/or" box and complicate the issues beyond the bumper-sticker morality with which both our culture and their prehistories had equipped them. These 16 students produced an aggregated total of 77 different moral concepts, which I collected and distributed to the class. The students finished the assignment with a realization that ethics will require much more of them than repeating a few hackneyed arguments and, more important, that ethical certainty is often elusive and always hard-won.

The most productive posture for ethics, as I emphasize in chapter 1, is a stance of not-knowing, a suspension of the idea that we already know what is right and good. Fruitful ethical inquiry begins with at least a grain of agnosticism. Nurturing a suspicion for the reassurances of certainty, displacing ourselves from this sort of comfort, is, likewise, what makes us more likely to approximate the moral truth.

While the need for certainty makes us vulnerable to moral absolutes and slogans, there is another reason we should be wary of moral certainty. Our moral perspective is grounded in our lives as temporal beings. All moral judgments are time-laden, inevitably "in place" in some specific temporal part of our ongoing lives. Usually we think of place as a spatial location, but it is also temporal, not just

Pascal's "true on this side of the Pyrenees, false on the other,"[18] but true at this time in the flux of my life. Merleau-Ponty gives a helpful description of this inextricable feature of human judgments:

> My hold on the past and the future is precarious, and my possession of my own time is always postponed until a stage when I may fully understand it, yet this stage can never be reached, since it would be one more moment, bounded by the horizon of its future, and requiring in its turn further developments in order to be understood.[19]

If there is no final point, no true resting place where the fabric of moral life is still, then making moral judgments must be accompanied by a deep humility. Moral judgments are tense (strained, taut, anxious) because they are laden with tense (past, present, future) in a systemic way. Every occasion for judgment has its own horizon of contingencies and uncertainties.[20] At a minimum, it should make us keenly sensitive to the need to displace our moral evaluations from any expectation of finality. To think otherwise is to assume the eternal perspective of a god.

At this point let me tie together a few threads of the discussion so far and anticipate a few more connections. What replaces the comforts of moral certainty are the learnings available to us as we embrace *un*certainty. Being uncertain is the only avenue to new knowledge, and thus acknowledgment of uncertainty is closely related to what I describe in chapter 1 as "Socratic ignorance." Yet embracing uncertainty requires a prior tolerance—a tolerance for moral ambiguity, that is, for appreciating that some moral truths will only gradually reveal themselves and are often hidden in the details and in the blind spots of the perspective from which we entertain an issue. The examples cited in the section of chapter 9 entitled "Cracking the Case" are useful illustrations of this point. In addition, the learnings of uncertainty and ambiguity are enabled by what I describe in the following discussion under the skill of "thinking slowly."

Emotional Skill: Learning from Our Feelings

Our emotional responses contain moral knowledge. Ethics requires us to notice what is happening in our hearts and our guts in various situations, especially those that make us uncomfortable. "Why does this issue—or this person—makes me uneasy or give me a flash of anger?" is an example of this kind of attention-giving. Of course, paying attention to our feelings does not mean giving them the final, authoritative voice in our judgments and choices, but rather puts us in a position to decide what sort of role they should have.

Many philosophical approaches have not considered feelings as a mode of ethical understanding. At best, they are considered of no value and, at worst, a genuine hazard to ethics. In this model of ethics, thoughts are trustworthy—because presumably they are subject to reason—whereas feelings just seem to well up in us; they are involuntary and thus irrational. When feelings become strong, this orthodoxy warns us, they are likely to lead us astray. This point of view permeates the history of Western ethics. Its roots can be traced at least as far back as Plato. In *Phaedrus*, Plato describes his tripartite view of the soul.[21] The highest form of the soul is the rational part, situated in the head, behind the eyes; its position at the top of the body surveying the field symbolizes its importance in governing the lower parts: the spirited soul, residing in the chest (the hearts and its emotions), and the appetitive soul, lying in the abdomen (with influence over eating and drinking) and in the groin area (the sexual appetites). In a healthy or well-ordered human life, Plato thought, the rational soul would exercise authority over the spirited and appetitive dimensions of a person. Leading an ethical life, according to this model, means following reason rather than giving the reins to emotions or appetites.

The Platonic discrediting of the emotions as sources of moral knowledge or authority has been a staple of most moral philosophy ever since and a chief ingredient in the teachings of Christianity, in which the precepts of divine revelation replace the ethical teachings of reason. Even if the governing force has changed from reason to revelation, the natural human emotions remain untrustworthy and morally suspect. The so-called seven deadly sins of Catholicism—pride, envy, anger, sloth, greed, gluttony, and lust—are typically interpreted as the result of perverted submission to the emotions or appetites. The Pauline writings of early Christianity and the teachings of St. Augustine, to take two notable and influential examples, are filled with worries about human emotions leading to sinfulness. This suspicion of emotion has been transmuted into worries about the precariousness of any ethical judgments that are based upon what Kant called human "inclinations."[22] There are, of course, counterexamples, for instance, in the writing of Nietzsche and the valorizations of human sentiments in the Scottish Enlightenment writings of David Hume and Adam Smith, but historically these voices express a minority position. Modern psychology and the writings of feminist thinkers have provided forceful corrective to this dualism of trustworthy reason/untrustworthy emotions, and I will address their contributions as I describe love as a primary moral concept in chapter 4.

Skill in ethical deliberation depends upon attention to our emotional life, especially an awareness of the way emotions can instruct us. First, emotions are instructive because they provide clues to the assets and liabilities of one's moral prehistory. Growing up in the rural and segregated South in the 1940s, 1950s, and 1960s, I had to learn not to be instinctively suspicious of people who were different. This was especially true for me regarding African Americans. I was in high school before I had black classmates. College experiences were another deep lesson in what I could learn from opening myself emotionally and intellectually to the life experiences of my black acquaintances. Black colleagues and lasting friendships came still later. Emotional responses are not just "how we happen to feel" but indicative of moral norms—for good, but also often for ill.

Second, and on the positive side, emotions are instructive in the sense that feeling compassion for others, or even just affinity with others, bespeaks a depth of human interconnectivity that eludes reason and logical processes. It is one thing to respect a noble ideal, such as the fundamental equality of persons, but the impetus to action comes from a felt response in the presence of another person. Without those feelings of connection, many of the ethical ideals to which reason leads us would have no motive force or staying power. In Jesus' parable, the Good Samaritan did not act on a moral ideal but was "moved by compassion" for the beaten man in the road.[23]

Buddhism teaches a helpful approach to human emotions. Rather than label emotions good or bad, Buddhism endorses a curiosity about them. The growing popularity of mindfulness adapts some of this Buddhist understanding. The idea is to become a witness to my feelings, rather than being captured by them and acting them out or trying to ignore them. Then I can decide whether they are toxic aspects of my prehistory I wish to change, or whether, alternatively, they are positively instructive and reinforcing to my moral ideals.

In a 1997 article Leon Kass coined the phrase "the wisdom of repugnance," an early expression of what we now call "the yuck factor."[24] Repugnance or disgust is not a moral argument, but it may well express a deep emotional wisdom. Such wisdom can be beyond our power to fully explain on rational grounds. For example, conceiving a child to create an organ donor for one's sick toddler may evoke a "yuck" response from some. For others, thinking of the suffering of pigs—how they are raised in confined and squalid conditions, pumped with antibiotics, and then killed for bacon and sausage—can call forth the revulsion of a "yuck" response. Kass's point is an important one. Deep feelings often carry a moral message of value beyond our powers to analyze fully. Still, examining critically what we find yucky may turn up misunderstandings or unrecognized biases. Yuck responses should above all make us curious and initiate an inquiry into why.

Cognitive Skill: Thinking Slowly

Most of the time we are required to think quickly, but not carefully. Quick thinking is the human default response. Ethics requires what Daniel Kahneman refers to as "System 2 thinking," the slower, less readily accessible form. Kahneman summarized his work in the 2011 book *Thinking, Fast and Slow*.[25] Just as "slow food" involves thoughtfully prepared and nourishing meals crafted from sustainable ingredients and stands in contrast to mass-produced, high-salt, and high-sugar "fast food," slow thinking involves deliberate, reflective, and critical assessment of one's own beliefs rather than reliance on largely unconscious and reactive thought processes. Fast thinking can be just as toxic as fast food. Kahneman argues that by understanding our inherent biases and questioning our intuitive beliefs, preferences, and initial impressions, we can limit the damage of bad judgments and decisions.

It will be obvious that what I have said about probing one's prehistory, our ignorance of some of our deepest moral values, relinquishing our moral vanity, and becoming a reflective witness to one's feelings all require slowing down. Ethical reasoning, like sound reasoning in all areas, requires a deliberate pacing. Among other things, ethical reasoning requires being clear-headed about assumptions and biases, weighing emotional responses, checking and rechecking facts, interpreting probabilities and outcomes, and sorting through a variety of stories about what our choices mean for ourselves and others. All this must precede choosing a principle of action and deciding. The potential flaws are numerous, which makes slow thinking essential. As Kahneman puts it, it is much easier for humans to think metaphorically than statistically. We have excessive confidence in what we think we know and a reluctance to acknowledge the full extent of our ignorance, as well as the uncertainty of the world we live in. We are prone to overestimate how much we understand.[26] To Kahneman's analysis I would add that we are prone to see our lives as justified and satisfying moral narratives. We overestimate our altruism and underestimate our selfishness. We frequently treat ourselves as the moral heroes of our storyline.

Consider the following situation. David McNeely was a retired professor. For more than 40 years he taught classics in a small liberal arts college and was a renowned instructor of Latin and Greek. At the point of his retirement he had a choice. His pension was structured so that he could take the full value of his pension, which would then end with his death, or he could take an amount reduced by 16 percent, which would continue for his spouse, Jane, were he to die first. He and Jane were the same age. Professors of Latin and Greek in small liberal arts colleges are not high wage earners, and even with the help of Social Security their income in retirement would be modest.

McNeely believed that Jane would precede him in death. Two years earlier, she had been diagnosed with early stage breast cancer that was treated with surgery and chemotherapy. While at this point there was no sign of recurrence, McNeely's first wife had died of breast cancer 10 years earlier, and he was resigned to the probability that he would lose Jane in the same way. "Just my fate," he confided to his friends.

The decision about which pension option to take seemed straightforward and quite clear to McNeely. He reasoned that he should maximize the income he and Jane could receive over whatever time they had left together, and he would continue to benefit from the same income after her demise. Without discussing the choice with Jane and against the advice of the pension fund management team, McNeely chose to receive the full benefit of his pension, which would end with his death. Three years later Jane was in good health with no recurrence of her cancer while McNeely was in the local inpatient hospice unit with only a few weeks to live. Jane outlived her husband by 17 years.

In retrospect, the flaws of quick reasoning in David McNeely's decision are easy to see. McNeely was wedded to a personal story line of tragically losing two spouses to the same disease. This fits the moral arc of a professor deeply schooled in the Greek tragic tradition. His devotion to this narrative overrode his weighing of the statistical probabilities. An otherwise healthy woman whose breast cancer is detected early and who is treated successfully has a survival expectation exceeding that of a healthy male of the same age. Here McNeely failed to look carefully at the data. Also important, McNeely had grown up in an impoverished family, and the nutritional deficits of his childhood and their compromising health effects in later life were not a part of his calculus. Here he simply didn't know what he didn't know. He failed to consider sufficiently his biases and the range of his ignorance and perhaps his own selfishness. He also did not give sufficient weight to the consequences of being wrong about which of them would survive the other. The moral flaw at work here is hubris. More time, more discussion, more probing and rethinking, more humility about the accuracy of his favored life narrative—more System 2 thinking—could have made his choice different and better.

I will return to the importance of reasoning carefully in the discussion of essential moral concepts in chapters 6 and 7, yet the most basic and important message is this: in ethics, take your time.

3
Basic Skills II

Imaginative Skill: Expanding the Reach of Our Empathy

Psychiatrist Richard Sobel describes empathy as "the ability of an individual to discern, both cognitively and emotionally, what another person is thinking or feeling at a particular moment in time."[1] Empathy thus defined always involves some distance between people. It is not a merging of feeling, nor is it exclusively emotional. What many think of as empathy, feeling what another person feels, Sobel refers to as sympathy. In sympathy we may laugh or cry spontaneously when others do so, in a kind of mirroring response. Sympathy, in this sense, is affective echoing. Empathy, by contrast, is a term indicating a more sophisticated, imaginative movement in which identity of feeling is not the core phenomenon, but in which imaginative insight is the key. The exercise of empathy allows for understanding another's thoughts and feelings without necessarily feeling them oneself. Empathy is the correct sense of what it must be like to walk in your shoes and to have the experiences you have. Sympathy is "I feel your pain" (when genuine and not a hackneyed effort to relate); empathy is "I can imagine what it must be like for you to have this pain." The object of empathy is an experience of another person—I do not have your experience, nor do I merge feelings with you—but your situation comes alive in my imagination and is respected and validated for what it is.

Studies have repeatedly shown that we are most likely to have natural empathy for people most like ourselves in age, sex, race, occupation, religious affiliation, and especially socioeconomic status.

The most difficult reaches of empathy are for those who differ from us on these indices. For example, white, middle-aged, professional males are likely to have little or no natural empathy for young black or Hispanic female workers who clean their offices. Why is this important? Because failures in empathy prohibit us from taking the moral perspectives of others into account. Rather, we are likely to dismiss them with labels and assumptions that imply that whatever moral perspectives they hold are likely inferior to our own. Lack of empathy cuts us off from serious listening. It treats others—those who look and act differently—as alien to us.

Empathy is not easy. It requires effort to try to imagine what another person is going through, and the lack of effort to understand is one of the more basic forms of disrespect. It says, "You are not worth knowing, not worth the effort to hear your views and see how they are rooted in your life experiences, just as mine are." It says, "I don't know how you size up your world morally, and it couldn't possibly matter to me. I can't imagine that you have anything to teach me." The repeated denial of empathy in one's life thus leads to an impoverished moral sensibility, one based on self-righteous pride and willful ignorance.

Here lies a point of significance. The nonempathic person is arrested from even the most elementary moves and insights of ethics. We do not stretch into imaginative recognition and emotional resonance with others just out of kindness, or because we are warm and sensitive people. We *must* do it if we are to learn—both about ourselves and about others. As social creatures, we are interactive mirrors for one another in a vast range of ways, some self-conscious, some not. I need a range of social interactions with diverse people to even have an accurate sense of who I am morally. So a fundamental question is: "With whom do I (or can I) empathize?" Some failures in ethics are cognitive failures, lapses in the logical application of principles, but more often ethical failures are lapses of empathic imagination, that is, a problem of narrow sentiments, a stunted or underdeveloped range of moral imagination.

The primatologist Frans de Waal puts it this way: "Our brain has been designed to blur the line between self and other. It is an ancient neural circuitry that marks every mammal, from mouse to elephant." On our good days humans can be as kind-hearted as bonobos and on our bad days as systematically cruel as chimps; we are the most "bipolar apes."[2] Empathy can lead to a higher form of moral life, greater skill in ethical reflection, and an enlarged capacity for kindness. But lack of empathy leads eventually to brutality. Sobel also makes much the same point and cites two modern authors, John Banville and Ian McEwan.

> In John Banville's novel *The Book of Evidence*, the protagonist explains how he came to senselessly murder a young woman: "This is the worst, the essential sin, I think, the one for which there will be no forgiveness: that I never imagined her vividly enough, that I did not make her live. Yes, that failure of imagination is my real crime, the one that makes the others possible. What I told the policeman is true—I killed her because for me she was not alive."[3]

Ian McEwan's *Atonement* carries the same message: "It wasn't only wickedness and scheming that made people unhappy, it was confusion and misunderstanding; above all, it was the failure to grasp the simple truth that other people are as real as you."[3]

A caveat here is important to forestall misunderstanding. Empathy is defined in a variety of ways, and many of these definitions make it synonymous with sympathy, or sameness of feeling with others. I oppose such a definition, in part because I think it is too shallow an understanding and in part because it tends to pit the emotions against reasoning as polar opposites, while in practical ethics the emotions and reason often work together. Moreover, following Sobel, I do not see empathy as an emotional skill, but as an imaginative one. From a practical point of view, all the skills discussed in this chapter and the previous one are important to ethics. Trying to determine which of them, if any, could be said to be the "foundation" for ethics—minimizing other capacities needed—is a wrong move and unimportant for how we routinely make our way in the world. For more on this point, see chapter 5, "Some Common Pitfalls," especially the section on the misguided search for foundations.

Assertive Skill: Claiming Our Own Moral Authority

This sounds deceptively simple, but it is a monumental leap to recognize and accredit oneself as a distinct moral authority and, eventually, the final moral authority for one's life. Like breaking from and reassessing the moral powers of one's prehistory, claiming moral power for one's self is a lifelong process. Part of the excitement of studying ethics is precisely this sort of individual self-recognition. It is a personal enlightenment that in some ways traces the Enlightenment period in Western thought.

The Enlightenment refers roughly to the period in seventeenth- and early eighteenth-century Western societies in which individualism, science, and reason ascended to become dominant modes of understanding the world and the human place in it. It marked a major transition away from monarchy and church traditions to representative governments and the validation of individual experiences in religion. In Germany, thinkers such as Kant and Goethe represented this shift; in France Voltaire and Rousseau are exemplars; in Scotland, Smith and Hume; and in England, Locke, Wollstonecraft, and Newton, along with many others. The emblem of the Enlightenment in America is nothing less than the founding of the United States, with representative thinkers such as Franklin, Jefferson, and Madison. Jefferson is an iconic figure in several areas, including constitutional government, religious freedom, and scientific progress. The inscription inside the dome at his memorial in

Washington, D.C., sums up the spirit of the Enlightenment: "I have sworn upon the altar of God eternal hostility against every form of tyranny over the mind of man."[4]

In his essay "What Is Enlightenment?" Immanuel Kant perhaps best summarizes the ethical impact of the Enlightenment.[5] The opening claim answers his question: "Enlightenment is man's emergence from his self-incurred immaturity." Note that he asserts that this immaturity is self-induced. It springs not from people's inability to think for themselves, or their lack of intellect, but their lack of courage. More specifically, Kant is urging his readers to use reason and judgment, breaking free from the censoring tutelage of others who pose as authorities over one's choices and sense of self. A contemporary way of saying this is, "Think for yourself." In other words, don't let other people do your thinking for you. Modern Western societies are not so subject to monarchies or church authorities as in the past, but our thinking can still be captured in many ways. For example, we are still prone to uncritically adopt the views of our families, friends, or religious, political, or other leaders, and the ascendency of social media over the past decade increases this risk. Think also of the current sophisticated forms of advertising, which are magnified by social media and the internet. Advertisers not only have infiltrated the Web but have collected a vast array of information about us, about our likes and dislikes, our shopping habits, our political views, our personal proclivities and opinions. The March 2018 news about the power of Cambridge Analytica and the Russian hackers to influence political processes by using the big data collected through social media platforms, such as Facebook, means that we can be subjected, unwittingly, to the authority of others in ways our forebears could not have imagined. Social media now sell private information to those who use the tools of behavioral economics and behavior politics, so that advertising is now better characterized as manipulation. This should not surprise us. Advertising is designed, after all, to alter our self-image and tie it to possession of a commercial product. Advertising that can use big data sets for subliminally influencing social values and shaping elections is a natural outgrowth.

One of the things important about the Kantian definition of Enlightenment is that it stresses not only vigilance about who is influencing us, but also courage to ask questions about ways we might be unwittingly subjected to the nefarious aims of others. Facebook, of course, and other social media platforms claim to provide an important social service, which makes questioning the unsavory aspects of their practices even more important. What was true for the great cultural movement of Kant's day is true for each of us now as we break first from the confines of our moral prehistories, but also from the increasingly sophisticated forms of moral and intellectual bondage that are so temptingly offered in the guise of community building and convenience. The overall message is more than "Think for yourself"; it is also "Be especially vigilant when those who may influence you claim to act from beneficent or socially desirable motives."

In stressing moral self-realization, I do not suggest that assertiveness and independence always bring an advance over one's early-life moral authorities or the accepted moral values in one's community. As discussed in chapter 1, we are capable of both moral progress and atrophy; we can grow better but also grow worse. The other skills discussed in this chapter and the previous one offer tests on what will count as a claim of moral authority that is an improvement rather than a decline. Whatever moral authority we claim for ourselves should never weaken the use of the other ethical skills discussed, nor cause us to ignore or pervert the concepts discussed in chapters 6 and 7. For example, an individual moral assertiveness that promotes my interests over those of the community, or that minimizes the suffering of others, or that arrogates to me special moral insights or privileges would be a sure sign of moral degradation rather than advancement.

Connective Skill: Linking Goodness and Happiness

It is a very old theme in ethics that good actions and attitudes promote or enhance happiness. Plato, Aristotle, Kant, Hume, Mill, and a wide range of other philosophers have asserted this thesis. What they meant by happiness differed, but for each, a well-lived, joyous life is not possible without adherence to ethical teachings. This is not, to be sure, a view universally shared. Thomas Hobbes, for example, writing during the English Civil War, believed that all human actions are at base self-interested, or ego-driven.[6] His view was that morality is just a public face we must put on because we lack the power to achieve our self-centered desires. The only happiness available in this mode of thinking is relief from not being robbed or killed. Still, most philosophers lack Hobbes's cynicism and believe there is an intrinsic connection between goodness and a happy life. This connection holds true for most theological doctrines as well, since they teach that human happiness in this life is deeply connected with orthodox beliefs and actions and not simply tied to the rewards of a blissful afterlife.

The old saw "Virtue is its own reward" expresses this deep connection between goodness and happiness for both philosophical and religious thought. It has a double meaning: first it indicates that one should not expect to become rich or famous by being a good person. And second, it means that virtuous practices teach a way of life that leads to a better kind of happiness, or as they typically say, true happiness—something more than the transitory satisfactions of acquiring material possessions, wielding more power, and drinking older whisky.

To clarify, an opportunistic reading of the connection between goodness and happiness might be something like this: "I want to be happy, and if being virtuous is the path to that end, I'll do it." Goodness is then reduced to the means to happiness, so that someone who might not otherwise have a motive to be virtuous now has one. It is like saying you find religious teachings stultifying, but you intend to adhere to these teachings anyway to gain a heavenly reward. This cynical reading neglects sincerity as an essential part of both moral virtue and religious belief. A calculation of rewards and punishments is not the right motivation for seeking to be good. To paraphrase Kant, it isn't enough to act in accord with the moral law. Virtue requires following the moral law out of respect for it, because one recognizes its fundamental motive force in one's thinking and doing. Hence Kant wanted to reserve the designation of "good" to a "good will."[7] More about Kant later. For now, the point is that virtue cannot be reduced to an instrumental value, another insight implied in the phrase "Virtue is its own reward."

The early twenty-first century has seen an outpouring of research on happiness. For example, the *Journal of Happiness Studies* says it is "devoted to scientific understanding of subjective well-being."[8] There is also a Happiness Research Institute that promotes happiness and studies that lead to happiness.[9] Prominently displayed on the Web are studies designed to change one's view of happiness, and many of them echo ancient philosophical and religious teaching. For example, they seem to show that more money doesn't lead to happiness (beyond a modest amount to meet one's needs), but happiness can be found through volunteering, being kind, smiling, and buying things for others (rather than oneself). More pointedly, gratitude and trust are cited as happiness producers.

We should be cautious in interpreting what all these studies mean, since it isn't clear what responders to these surveys on happiness meant when they said that these activities and attitudes improve their happiness. And are the researchers who conduct these studies suggesting that their results can be used in an instrumental, self-help way as previously discussed—for example, just smile and be kind, because it will make you happier? That said, it is always possible that one can initially smile and be kind from an instrumental and self-serving motive and find that, over time, one is genuinely smiling and being kinder out of altruistic motives. Practices, even those undertaken with ulterior motives, can change people. If I smile and practice kindness over time I may be changed in the process into a person for whom these activities have intrinsic worth. So, I might say, "Yes, I began doing these things because I simply wanted to be happier. And now I find that I do them because that's just who I am." In this last quote being good and feeling good, being good and the pleasure of self-esteem, are now intimately connected.

What kinds of things make us happy? The teachings of ethics are that there are levels or kinds of happiness and that these can be graded from lower to higher. Some forms of happiness we seem to share with animals and some are distinctive to humans; some are transient and some more durable; some engage our appetites and some our desires for power and fame, while others bespeak the achievement of our moral potential. Ethics can teach us a distinctive form of happiness. Aristotle spoke of this as *eudaimonia*, best translated as "flourishing"—realizing one's potential for excellence, including moral excellence, as a human being.[10]

Ethics as a human activity depends on at least some reflective grasp of the inextricable tie between being happy, in the more refined sense, and being good.

Narrative Skill: Story-Making at Intersecting Life Trajectories

Humans are storytelling creatures, but more important, we are *story-creating* creatures.[11] Every ethics case is a shorthand story, constructed by someone. Each one offers a narrative that describes the facts in the larger setting of a decision, usually with assumptions about the motives and intentions of the moral agents involved. Every ethics narrative constructs a flow from moral tension through moral analysis and deliberation to discernment, to some culminating judgment and action. I will have more to say about the construction of ethics cases in chapter 9. Here my focus is on the skill, and hazards, of ethics narration.

Hospital ethics consultations are particularly rich venues for knotty ethical problems, and story construction is a central feature of these cases. But in any setting—business, legal, political, or medical—and for any deliberative process, the same narrative ingredients are always in play: interpreting facts, discerning motives and assessing the appropriate roles of moral agents, assigning responsibilities, and constructing an integrated stream of possibilities. And because the moral arcs of any two lives, at any given point in time, are never the same, no two people ever engage this storying process from the same angle of entry. This complexity of story-making within intersecting life narratives is seldom discussed but of great importance. Failure to pay attention to it leads to the easy assumption that we all feel and think the same things—in other words, to homogenization of moral experiences, superficial categorizations, labeling, and often to moral dogma.

Here I offer a case from my own clinical ethics consultation experiences. As an ethics consultant I am inevitably a story-maker. In this role, skepticism about my own interpretations is just as important as skepticism about the reliability of any of the other storytellers on the scene. I invite you to consider the responsibilities that emerge once we acknowledge that we must inevitably construct moral narratives and that such narratives intersect with other people in their own unique moral life trajectory.

> *A resident physician in the surgical ICU called at 8:00 AM requesting an ethics consult. According to his brief history, the patient, Mr. Henry Bush (this and all case names are pseudonyms), 78 years old with a 10-year history of Alzheimer's dementia, was admitted a week ago following an unimpeded fall on his face from a standing position. He was at home at the time, cared for by his daughter, Sara Bush. The patient was taking Plavix (an anticlotting prescription medication) at the time of his fall, which exacerbated the bleeding and complicated*

his injuries. Surgical intervention following hospital admission was unsuccessful, and Mr. Bush remains intubated and unresponsive following the surgery. In the judgment of the attending surgeon and the consulting neurologist, further intervention will not repair his brain injuries or restore Mr. Bush to consciousness. An aggressive course of care may soon require a PEG (percutaneous endoscopic gastrostomy, or feeding tube), and the medical team is reluctant to place it, given the very poor prognosis. However, discussion with the spouse and the daughter are going nowhere. The spouse also suffers from dementia, of less severity than the patient's, but she is clearly unable to act as Mr. Bush's surrogate. Sara, the only child, in her mid-fifties, is the appropriate surrogate for Mr. Bush, but she refuses to discuss palliative care and comfort-only measures as an option. The difficulty of communicating effectively with the daughter and disagreement about the goals of care are the primary reasons the resident gives for the ethics consult request.

Having read the information in the EMR (electronic medical record), I arrived in the surgical ICU about an hour after the initial consult request. I had brief conversations with the resident and the bedside nurse that confirmed my general understanding of the situation. As I approached Mr. Bush's room, it was clear that the patient's daughter, Sara Bush, was in an intense conversation with the attending physician, who was describing the patient's situation, the very poor prognosis and why comfort-only measures were—in her view—important to consider now. The daughter was having none of it, saying it was "too early to think about that," and insisting that her father needed a chance to recover. The physician saw me approach but did not signal for me to enter the conversation. I remained outside the room but within earshot. One feature of their conversation struck me—that the physician interrupted the daughter as she was speaking, correcting her impressions about her father's condition and citing the evidence of computed tomography (CT) scans and other technical metrics of prognosis. The interruptions were not unkind but were repetitive. Ten minutes later, as the attending left the patient's room, I walked with her down the hallway. She thanked me for coming and said the daughter doesn't seem to realize how dire the situation is, indicating that what I had overheard was one of several (unsuccessful) attempts to reconsider the goals of care. Given this patient's age, compromised health, and the extent of his injuries, there was nothing—either in the collective memory of the ICU team or in the literature—to suggest that a recovery was a realistic possibility. "I never say 'never,'" she said. "But this case is about as clear as it gets. Maybe you can help here."

Even at this very early stage in the consult, at least three narratives are in play. The EMR itself is a narrative, really a variety of narratives, in the forms of daily progress notes from physicians, nurses, respiratory therapists, and others; consult notes from neurology; several fragments of social history; and other slivers of information with varying degrees of relevance, most requiring discernment and interpretation to build a coherent picture. A second distinct narrative is the story of why this case has come to be categorized as an ethical concern for the medical team, as expressed in terms of the daughter's inability or perhaps unwillingness to hear a discouraging prognosis and the resulting frustration of the professional caregivers.

A third narrative is the tentative sketch running through my mind as a consultant—partly factual, partly anticipatory and conjectural, inevitably personal—about what is going on here. So far, I have received a call, read the medical record, talked with three of the professional caregivers, and overheard a conversation with the patient's daughter. These are fragments at best. Yet the story forming in my mind is inevitably influenced by a wide range of persons and experiences I have brought with me to this consult. Among these are not only other physicians, patients, and families I have worked with in the past and the hospital and death experiences of previous consultations, but also my memories of the care-trajectories and deaths of both of my parents and some of my friends; my work

40 years ago as a minister; and a range of experiences with such human phenomena as hope, denial, grief, what people do in a crisis, and the beneficial and toxic uses of moral and spiritual resources. In short, my internal story elements are complex and idiosyncratic, and at least some of these elements lie at a tacit level of awareness most of the time.

To assist with resolving the case, the next obvious conversation needed to be with the daughter, who has, with brief respites, kept vigil at her father's bedside since his admission. Through my initial conversation with her, several signposts marking the terrain of her story became evident. She is an only child, is single, and feels a deep sense of obligation to her parents; a year ago she moved nearby from another state to take care of them. After a year she is now experienced in the hard, daily work of caregiving. And her tone indicates she may well feel some responsibility for her father's predicament. Although she did not say so explicitly, her father fell "on her watch."

A second marker in the daughter's narrative is that until recently, she worked professionally with rehabilitating children with injuries. Not only did she physically move her residence to care for her aging parents, she also gave up a career in her mid-fifties to satisfy these filial duties. Given her knowledge of rehabilitation processes, she felt she had some warrant to speak about her father's prognosis. And yet her experience was entirely with children, none of whom were as severely compromised as Mr. Bush. (A bedside nurse later explained that she had discussed the differences in prognosis between injuries in children and trauma in the elderly with the daughter several times, but with no sense of uptake.)

A third and more complex narrative turn was that Mr. Bush had completed advance care planning. He had both a living will and a durable power of attorney for health care. On Mr. Bush's admission the daughter had indicated the presence of these documents but kept them in her possession. As her father's condition had worsened, she decided not to show them to the healthcare team, or talk about their contents, for fear they would be used against her and compromise her father's care. "I wish they could be shredded," she said. She refused to give them to me as well. She was willing, however, to let me read them in her presence, but not to make copies.

They were the standard advance care planning forms, duly executed, with signatures of witnesses in place and properly notarized. The initials of Mr. Bush were scratched into his signature line. The intent of the documents was clear: to forgo life-sustaining treatment in situations just like this. What to make of the authenticity of such a document from a person with progressed Alzheimer's disease became the new puzzle within the old one. The date on the forms was barely a year ago. Moreover, the durable power of attorney named the spouse as the surrogate, and she had already been informally disqualified by the healthcare team as able to act in this capacity. "Do you think this is an accurate indication of your father's wishes?" I asked. "No," she replied, "I don't think he knew what he was doing, and I am sorry we ever did this." "We all hope for improvement," I said, "but it may not happen. Do you think your dad would want to be sustained in his current state?" Her reply startled me. "People are waiting on him here. He always liked being waited on. He enjoyed that sort of attention."

Sometimes the rituals of caring persist even when the acts of caring have no conscious recipient, no possibility of being knowingly received as care. That seemed very likely here. Yet in the presence of caring, interrogation of its logic can seem out of place. So I decided, rightly or wrongly, not to probe further with the next obvious question: "What if he is not able to experience being waited on? Would that count?" I couldn't find it in me to pose this further question to her, one I would have immediately launched toward graduate or medical students. There is educational value to ethics consultations, but this woman was not my student, and she had trusted me with information she had denied to others. More important, she had entrusted me with some of her story, a narrative that whatever else I made of it, I could not ignore or discount. In that 50-minute conversation she had ceased to be a "case" or a "problem family member in denial," and become a real person. I had, in the middle of our conversation, begun to call her "Sara."

I then silently considered a worrisome set of questions—a private sidebar narrative. Should I ask the daughter her permission to reveal the contents of the advance care planning documents to the healthcare team? Or as an advocate of "best care" for this patient, was it my responsibility to speak with the professional caregivers with or without her permission? Would the clinicians find in these documents too easy a confirmation of the course of action they thought most advisable? Most ethics consultants can recount many cases in which advance care planning documents were ignored by family, sometimes because they disagree with them, sometimes because it feels like giving up, and sometimes because their courage fails, despite their best intentions. By failing to discuss my findings with the healthcare team, was I becoming complicit in yet another such family failure to honor what the patient wanted? Would these advance care documents now simply be irrelevant, given the patient's prognosis? And if relevant, did they have a shred of validity? After a pause I asked the daughter, "You are facing such a tough decision here. Can I discuss the contents of these documents with the medical team? I think it may be helpful to them and perhaps also to you." "OK," she said, to my surprise and relief. The relevance of these documents, or lack of it, could now become an explicit part of any future conversations, making communication more transparent.

At this point I took my leave, and following instinct rather than protocol, I said, "God bless you." My own theological convictions are too skeptical to imply any concrete meaning to this departing gesture, but something about crisis and habit seem to eke this phrase out of me in consult work. More than anything, perhaps, it's a token of empathy and regard for a fellow human being.

Simply being an auditor to Sara's story and participating in this modest interaction with her placed me in a changed relationship with her. Knowing even a few parts of her larger story, I couldn't ignore them. The poverty of principled ethics, when taken alone, is that they flatten out this fragile sense of belonging to, protecting, and honoring another person's story. When they flatten narratives of care, the loss is even more damaging. Even if I might choose differently for my own parents (in fact, I have), I now knew something of who this daughter was in relation to her own father, how her sense of helping him now at the margins of his life was ultimately rooted in her love for him, and how her sense of self was grounded in that affection. This rootedness does not, of course, make her choices "right," but beneficent motivation should always, at least, give us pause in thinking we know better. To approach the medical team about the advance care documents without her permission would have been in some sense to betray her. It also would have been to betray whatever sense of his own well-being her father might have held, influenced as he likely was by her care for him over the last year and, indeed, by her concern for him over many years of her adult life. Narrative is a profound mode for understanding ethics not because it resolves problems, but because it forces us to attend to the human voices, including our own, behind what is being said.

I am acutely aware that this is my story, told from my point of view of an ethics consultant, with certain framing assumptions and agendas. This story is also colored and shaped by my own history, both professional and personal, intersecting with the stories of others in this situation. As such I am hesitant to declare the outcome good or bad, successful or unsuccessful, regarding the problems that occasioned my being called. I think and hope that my presence improved communication, and that is an inherent good as well as an instrumental one. But whether and how my presence improved decision-making is an open question. I am also agnostic about whether the "best care" for Mr. Bush was realized. "Best" always presupposes some goal, and goals are a function of which narratives are accredited and affirmed.

In this case the daughter's narrative was dominant, and so within a few days Mr. Bush received a PEG and a tracheostomy and was discharged to a long-term, acute care facility. While it was very unlikely that this course of action was harmful to Mr. Bush in terms of physical pain, it may have been harmful to his dignity—a matter on which he, regrettably, could not speak. It was also very likely a societal harm in terms of the costs incurred for his continuing care. Some, including members of the ICU team, might count this as a failure, but I think this judgment presumes too much. My hope was that with a little more time Sara Bush was able to let her father go. Ethics consultants are typically denied access to resolution of situations after discharge because we work for institutions and not patients or their families, nor for society at large. But whatever the outcome, an attitude of robust pluralism in ethics seems best. Ethics is not like finding universally correct answers in the back of the math book. It is more like muddling through, doing what is possible, and often trying to find the least harmful alternative in tragic situations. Indeed, the point of being aware of the power of multiple, intersecting narratives in any morally charged situation is to resist the temptation to adopt a privileged position that assumes that I know what is best, or even that I know the right ethical methods or processes for each situation. Ethics consultation—like being helpful whatever one's role—is usually an effort to help others to locate, interrogate, and finally to trust their own moral resources and to seek some measure of convergence with the other stakeholders.

Since as moral actors we are never free from a narrating role and its interpretive task, humility is always needed, always a virtue. The humility is twofold: there is the humility in creating or constructing a moral narrative to make sense of the issue at hand, and there is also the humility required as I realize that my tale of moral sensemaking intersects with others, each with his or her own story, and each person is—as am I—working to discern the meaning of this issue within the moral arc of their lives.

4
Exercises Using the Skills

Nineteen Exercises in Eight Groupings

In chapters 2 and 3, I describe a core set of skills needed for ethics. In this chapter, I offer a set of prompts designed to probe our understanding and use of those capacities.[1] These prompts are grouped under eight headings and address the following: curiosity about one's moral sensibility; broad empathy; conceptual agility; identifying emotional registers; sensitivity to suffering; moral certainty/uncertainty; moral authority; and happiness. The prompts under each heading seek to get at the same capacity in a different way.

These exercises are not a measure of ethics per se. The true test for ethics is choices and actions over one's life history, the moral arc of a life, not verbal or written responses at a point in time. The benefit from the exercises is greater clarity about the shape of one's moral sensibility and a capacity to reflect more critically and deeply. The prompts do not ask for a discussion of specific good or bad choices we may have made; they focus on the abilities that enable and inform ethical reflection and deliberation.

I recommend responding to these prompts orally first and then in writing. The writing process usually brings out more details and undiscovered features. Try doing the exercises in pairs or with three people, with each person taking turns being the responder to the prompt and then the listener who voices the follow-up. When three are involved, the third person serves as the silent auditor of the other two participants. Responders should be given a few minutes to gather their thoughts, since the prompts ask for things we do not routinely think about. Each person in the pair or threesome can give an assessment along the lines outlined below. Again, the objective is not to judge good or bad, right or wrong, but to consider and weigh one's agility with the human skill evoked by the prompt. While these exercises are focused on responses to the prompts, careful listening and providing thoughtful feedback to others' responses are also skills essential to ethics.

Curiosity about One's Moral Sensibility

1. Most of us have *short sayings*—reminders, aphorisms, words of wisdom, little mantras—that we say to ourselves when we are considering a moral issue. What are yours, and how do they work for you?
   Follow-up: Describe when and how you learned them.
2. Sometimes, when we consider a difficult moral situation, we *feel* that one possible decision would be good or right, even while we *reason* that a different decision would be good or right. Describe a situation in which you experienced such an internal divergence or conflict.
   Follow-up: What does this tell us about the nature of ethics? How did you resolve the issue you describe?
3. Most of us remember experiences about which we would say, "That was an occasion in which I grew morally," a time when we experienced a broadening of our ethical horizons or saw that the moral dimensions of life are more expansive than we had previously thought. Describe one such experience you have had.
   Follow-up: Who were the central figures in this experience? What role did they play?

Broad Empathy

1. Most of us have been in situations in which we realized it was important to *try to see things from another person's point of view*. Describe a situation in which you realized it was important to try to see things from another person's perspective.
   Follow-up: How successful were you in your effort? What made it difficult to entertain the other person's perspective?
2. We often find ourselves in situations in which it is difficult to *empathize with people who are different from us*. For example, differences in age, race, social class, or life priorities can make it more difficult to empathize with another person. Talk about a time when differences between yourself and another person made it difficult for you to empathize with that person.
   Follow-up: What did you learn from making this effort?
3. Name a book, film, poem, play, etc. that showed you the importance of *imagining the lives of others*. Describe what it was like when you realized how important it can be to imagine others' lives.
   Follow-up: How has this experience with the book, film, poem, play, etc. continued to affect your thinking?

Conceptual Agility

1. Each of us has practical, *working understandings of key ethical concepts or ideals, such as truthfulness or conscience* that orient us, help us keep our feet morally, or help us make decisions we can live with and respect. Select one concept that is important to you and describe a situation in which it came into play.
   Follow-up: When and how did you learn this concept or ideal?

2. Most of us have had an experience in which we initially adopted a strong position on some moral issue, but at some later point *found ourselves supporting an opposing position* (or at least a very different one). Describe a time when this happened to you.

   Follow-up: Did this change take place over time, or do you remember a particular experience that led to this change of perspective?

3. Sometimes people undergo experiences that teach them *new meanings of ethical ideals they have always held*, ideals such as compassion, kindness, forgiveness, or service. Describe an experience in which a cherished ideal took on new meaning for you.

   Follow-up: How did the new meaning differ from your previous understanding?

Identifying Emotional Registers

1. Describe a difficult time in your life when you tried to *block out your emotional responses*. Were you successful in this, or did your emotions override your control or reemerge at a later time? What moral learning does this experience carry?

   Follow-up: Would you, in general terms, describe your attitude toward your emotions as trusting, guarded, curious, or, just what?

2. Describe a time in which you began to realize that your *emotional responses toward yourself or others could be moderated or changed*? What was going on in your life at the time?

   Follow-up: What do you consider the most influential sources of this flexibility in emotional response? Perhaps your family of origin, your friendships, or your spouse or long-term partner?

3. Name a person you consider *emotionally resilient*, that is, able to recover or adjust from emotionally taxing or potentially damaging events. Briefly narrate this person's story, as you understand it.
    Follow-up: How does emotional resilience affect the rest of a person's moral life, in terms of future actions and choices?

Sensitivity to Suffering

1. When thinking about *suffering*, most of us think first about *pain*. Yet people can suffer in many ways. Describe a situation in which you witnessed suffering that is best described in terms other than pain, or as something more than pain.
    Follow-up: How might this broader understanding of suffering be helpful in your personal or professional life?
2. Most of us at some point *witness someone suffering and then later find that it is difficult to talk about that person's suffering*. Think of an instance in which you witnessed another suffer in a way you found difficult to discuss. How has this experience affected your understanding of suffering?
    Follow-up: How might such experiences relate to your current or future personal life? How might such experiences relate to your professional life?

Moral Certainty/Uncertainty

1. Describe a conversation in which you began with *a sense of certainty* about some ethical question/issue and then, in the course of the conversation, you began to doubt or question your previous convictions.
    Follow-up: Was this a single conversation or a series? Did it involve one person or several? What did you feel when you moved from more to less certain?

2. Most of us are uncomfortable with *ambiguity*, that is, with situations that admit to multiple interpretations or meanings, since these situations leave us uncertain about how to respond. For example, sometimes it is hard to tell whether remarks about us or others are compliments or insults. A reference letter I once received on a prospective employee said, "If you can get this person to work for you, you'll be a lucky man." In medical care the application of a life-saving therapy may truly help patients or be ineffective and simply add to their suffering. Describe a situation of ambiguity from your own experience.

   Follow-up: How long were you able to leave the situation you describe unsettled? Can you describe the moral advantages and disadvantages of allowing ambiguous situations or events to settle without forcing a conclusion?

Moral Authority

1. Describe a time when you knew you were *in charge of your own moral life*, a time when you knew that regardless of what anyone else thought, your moral values are something you were responsible for.

   Follow-up: What was going on in your life at the time? Was the feeling that accompanied this experience one of apprehension or liberation?

2. We all have *moral heroes or heroines*, people who we think have exhibited some moral trait, such as courage or compassion, in a special way. Who comes to mind for you? What makes that person exemplary?

   Follow-up: Describe a specific episode from this hero's or heroine's life that manifested her or his exemplary quality. Why might others *not* think of that person as exemplary?

Have your heroes and heroines changed over time? What do you think accounts for this change?

Happiness

1. Describe three occasions on which you have known happiness. Does *the sense of happiness seem different or the same* in these three occasions?

   Follow-up: Can the kinds of happiness you have described be graded or evaluated into short-term or long-term, more or less fitting or appropriate, etc.?

2. Describe a situation in which you felt that someone (perhaps yourself) was *happy for the wrong reasons* or was feeling happy in a way that was not fitting.

   Follow-up: What accounts for this inappropriate happiness? What response, if not happiness, do you think would have been appropriate to the situation and person you have described?

Assessing Responses

Inadequate responses are those in which you are befuddled by the question or in which, on reflection, you now see your response as clichéd or hackneyed, showing little or no insight into the topic.

Adequate responses are relevant and on topic but lack details or show less insight into how the experience contributed to your moral development. Merely adequate responses will lack the authenticity, specificity, or degree of insight characteristic of the best responses.

Best responses narrate a concrete experience (including details that add to the experience's authenticity) and demonstrate insight into how the experience shaped your perspective or encouraged moral growth. Responses at this level typically show facility with one or more of the skills and conceptual tools. Frequently such responses evoke curiosity about the shape of your moral life and that of others.

5
Some Common Pitfalls

Ethics can go wrong in a wide range of ways. Neglecting the skills described in chapters 2 and 3, or ineptly practicing them, is one place to start in cataloguing the difficulties. Failure to understand the conceptual tools in chapters 6 and 7 is another potential problem source. Any of these factors, and more, can be at work when ethics goes wrong. Five hazards are especially pertinent:

- The trap of either/or thinking—a simplistic understanding of ethical choices;
- Expecting too much from theory—overestimating the importance of theory and undervaluing the insights of practice;
- The desire for a unifying definition of ethics—the misguided search for foundations;
- Restricting what experiences have ethical weight—truncating the sources of moral discernment; and
- Treating mysteries as moral problems—failing to acknowledge the limits of ethics.

The Trap of Either/Or Thinking

Consider the following case as presented by Benjamin Freedman.[1]

Mrs. A is a 68-year-old woman with colon cancer, with metastatic liver involvement and a mass in the abdomen. She is not expected to survive longer than a few months. Other than a course of antibiotics and palliative care, no active treatment is indicated or planned. She is alert and knows she has an infection, but her family refuses to inform her of the cancer diagnosis and asks the medical team not to tell her.

There are several ways we might approach this situation. One relies on *utility* as the primary operating principle: concealing her diagnosis is wrong because it leads to undesirable results; she will eventually learn (or has already guessed) her condition; and concealment also makes it difficult for the medical and nursing staff and is generally bad policy because if widely practiced it could undermine public trust in doctors.

But one could also reason to the same conclusion using a duty-oriented principle: concealing her diagnosis is wrong because she has a right to this information. No matter what her family wants, and regardless of the consequences, there is a duty to disclose. A third, virtue-based approach might employ the following reasoning: "Being a physician means that I must be truthful with my patients." Or perhaps, "Patients depend on physicians to have the honesty and prudence to know *what* to tell them and *how much* to tell them about their diagnosis and prognosis." In this last interpretation, the medical virtues of honesty and prudence shape the decision.

All three of these possible responses presume that telling the patient of her diagnosis is the right course. Yet a utilitarian, a duty-oriented, or a virtue-oriented case can also be made for withholding the information, as the family wants. Withholding information would likely rely on the principle of not harming the patient, at least in the short run, or on the virtue of willing the good for this patient, under the assumption that she would be harmed by knowing the cancer diagnosis. Modern readers may detect a taint of paternalism with the latter course of action, since we are taking the family's notion of what is good as overriding and definitive.

Note that we are left at this point with a rather typical either/or, to disclose the diagnosis or not, as the stark and exhaustive sum of the available choices. What third choice could there be?

In his article about this case, Benjamin Freedman reminds us that in many situations there are more than two choices, and an important part of ethics is having enough intellectual agility to imagine what the additional options might be. Freedman says, basically, let's give the choice to the patient about how much she is told. Here is a path that would capture this third alternative: we ask the patient just how she would like to have information about her care handled, especially the diagnostic and prognostic information, including alternative therapies. Would she like to be told these things herself, or would she prefer that these matters be handled by the family? To be sure, this question must be addressed to her when the family is out of the room to reduce any implicit coercive influence on her response. The genius of this third alternative is that it honors her autonomy, at a higher level than just giving her the facts. It allows her to be her own moral agent or to choose a proxy who will carry the burden of decisions. The third alternative also treats her beneficently, since it refrains from providing information to her that may be unwelcome. She gets to decide what and how much she wants to know. This is but one example of moving out of the entrapment of either/or to a third and more appropriate course of action. Almost every situation admits to a third option. If one isn't obvious, it's time to get creative.

Expecting Too Much from Theory

Ethical theories constitute an important part of our moral toolkit. Theories provide a more systematic and consistent way to consider our choices. Consider the choices presented above regarding Mrs. A, the 68-year-old woman with metastatic cancer. The theories sketched in this case—utilitarianism, a duty ethic, and a virtue approach—provided three possible scaffolds for analyzing the alternatives. Theories generate principles, which help us see the moral values at play in our decisions and actions. Just so, utilitarianism helps us consider the various forms of happiness that might result to Mrs. A and her family in alternative scenarios, a duty ethics helps us consider which actions would respect Mrs. A as a person, and a virtue-oriented approach centers on what character traits should be dominant for the doctor. Principles can also have a powerful corrective function. If, for example, we believe very strongly in the principle of respecting rights, we will eventually see that this principle will lead us to recognize rights in novel and unexpected places, such as the rights of transgender persons, or the rights of endangered species. The expanded application of principles into new and often unforeseen venues is a major force for moral progress.

Yet theoretical approaches to ethics, and the principles they spawn, require careful use. For example, we sometimes fall in love with a favored principle and use it when other principles would be better, or at least have a modulating effect. The welfare and happiness of children might require that they all be vaccinated for the typical childhood diseases. Yet mandatory vaccination based on this utilitarian mandate would run roughshod over the rights of parents to raise their children as they see fit. Here, at a minimum, some balancing of theories and principles is required.

If multiple theories can be useful, how do we know which theory or theories are most germane? One way to discern the answer is by recognizing that every ethical theorist has a particular view of the human situation and assumptions about which tendencies are likely to lead us astray. For example, here is Kant's summary of the generic human moral struggle to which his ethics speaks: "The human being feels within himself a powerful counterweight to all the commands of duty, which reason presents to him as so deserving of the highest respect—the counterweight of his needs and inclinations, the entire satisfaction of which he sums up under the name 'happiness.'"[2]

Hence, if I feel disinclined to listen to the voice of duty and attend instead to my own needs and inclinations, Kant's theory may be quite helpful. Alternatively, if my moral situation inclines me to presume too much control, I would do well to heed the advice of the Stoic philosopher Epictetus, whose portrait of the human moral dynamic begins with a sharp distinction between what is in my control (very little), and what is not.[3]

In brief, the extent of the usefulness of any ethical theory is the extent to which we see the portrait of the human moral struggle that theory presupposes as correct, or applicable to us, in our current situation. One of the reasons multiple ethical theories are needed is that human moral experiences are not just of one type, for example, duty versus inclinations or tendencies of excessive control versus a more realistic account of our powers. Sometimes duties conflict with other duties; at other times our good intentions become problematic because they make us prone to meddling rather than helping. There is no such thing as the standard moral perplexity to which a single theory will always give us the right resolution.

Moreover, our tendencies and experiences change as we change. Theories and the principles they endorse that were truly important to me in my late teens became less relevant to me in late middle age and seem remote from my concerns in my early seventies. For example, as a young adult intent on establishing my independence, the notions of freedom and autonomy were very appealing. In later life within a family and as a professional working with colleagues, solidarity, interdependence, and loyalty came to the fore as moral concepts I routinely needed. As I age, independence is once again quite important, but now less as breaking away and self-realization and more as a sustaining of physical and mental functioning. Also, I now find I have an appreciation for routine kindness that eluded me earlier.

Again, theories typically highlight single moral principles, often ones of great importance, yet most of the genuine conundrums, both socially and personally, do not lend themselves to simple, single-principle solutions. Moral issues typically exceed and outrun the capacity of our best theories and our most cherished principles. Or put another way, moral experiences are more diverse and complex than the theories in which we try to encapsulate and explain them. Theorizing seldom keeps the inadequacy of theory to practice in view. The best use of theories and the principles they provide is not as grand sweeping solutions, but as potentially useful tools. Keeping lots of instruments in the ethics toolkit is an essential part of not falling prey to a single theoretical system.

In addition, theoretically sponsored principles sometimes have a more limited application than anticipated. Modern feminist researchers and writers have been especially attentive to the way the dominant ethical theories flounder in accounting for specific, concrete moral experiences. For example, consider the groundbreaking psychological studies of Carol Gilligan. In 1982 Gilligan published her research on the moral development of women, in a book titled *In a Different Voice*.[4] She claimed that females tend to see moral problems in terms of relationships. They are prone to think of their choices in problem-solving as issues of care and responsibility for those relationships. By contrast, males tend to see moral problems in terms of rules and principles and are prone to think of their choices as logical adjudications. Women's moral orientations tend toward valuing and preserving ties among persons, while men tend toward abstract thinking by an agent largely removed from and impartial to the parties involved. Gilligan's claim is not that there are precise gender types for moral experience but that the model of the moral self as an isolated and principled thinker is insufficient and needs to be balanced by a more relational model.

The implications of Gilligan's research for our understanding of moral theory are substantial. Her research directly challenges the adequacy of thinking of any theory as providing principles or maxims that can simply be applied to cases. Her work suggests that past theories, especially those of the Enlightenment, presuppose a single and unencumbered agent rather than a person grounded in complex relationships that shape our understandings of ourselves. Moral problems can no longer be formulated as if the agent were essentially solitary and could contemplate the scope of his or her duties from afar. The self is already and, essentially, immersed in a web of relationships and their attendant responsibilities. The ethical formulations of many theories exhibit precisely the hierarchical distancing and the assumption of optional relationships depicted in the "male" model. Attending to the second and different voice in moral experience would mean moving ethics beyond reliance on applying a principle to problem cases and then expecting a solution. All moral judgments must then be understood as relevant to and evident in the ongoing, everyday activities of persons in their webs of work, friendship, and family life.

This is not to say that theoretical considerations are always wrong or not needed. Theories constitute an important way to step back and reflect on assumptions and implications in how we frame moral problems. The problem comes when we see theorizing as the definitive move in ethics, making theoretical cogency the final arbiter of the goodness or rightness of actions, instead of being one tool among others that helps us think. Theorizing is often a useful exercise, but it is only one kind of reflective activity among many. Theories are not necessarily more important than storytelling, talking with friends, imagining alternatives, meditating, praying, singing, and a host of other activities, all of which can provide reflective perspective. The family with a comatose loved one in the medical intensive care unit (ICU), facing a life-or-death decision, whose deliberative process includes taking a long walk, praying with the ICU staff, talking to a trusted neighbor, or telling stories about their ill relative does no worse—and often better—than those families who decide by mapping the options on a decision tree of utilities.

On a concrete, personal level, my experience has been that the love of theory has a debilitating effect. When I go to theory, I tend to stop listening. Of course, I still understand the words people are speaking, but I stop attending to the way their words are gestures pointing toward their constellation of values. Instead I hear these words as successful or unsuccessful candidates for fulfilling the requirements of my theory. The real resolution of moral problems is always practical, not theoretical. Ethics, finally, is never concerned simply with theories; it is concerned with what we are doing—and what we think we are doing—as we navigate through the choices that life presents.

The Desire for a Unifying Definition of Ethics

Implicit in what I have said so far is that there is no Ur-form, no foundational idiom for ethics, and no essential normative shape for how to analyze our moral sensibilities. We can read the history of modern Western philosophy as a series of efforts to finally locate the definitive form for ethics, either in duties, or in utilities, or in virtues and vices, and so on. Yet it is evident to many—although certainly not all—that the efforts to find one final definitive form for all the moral concerns of our species in an overarching and complete theory is a Procrustean exercise. Procrustes, in the mythology of ancient Greece, was a king who, following a sumptuous meal, invited his guests to spend the night. But he cut or stretched his guests to fit the bed he provided, putting short guests on a rack to stretch them out and chopping off the feet of others who were too tall. Hence, a Procrustean approach to ethics involves either stretching moral experience or reducing it to fit the favored approach, in both cases disfiguring it to fit the requirements of a single definition. Charles Taylor has described this well in asserting that "the ethical is not a homogeneous domain, with a single kind of good, based on a single kind of consideration."[5]

My experience suggests that pluralism in the domain of ethics is not superficial but deep and multifaceted. It is not just that moral experience is not of a single type. Nor is ethics the function of, or a capacity held by, a single human ability. The skills described in chapters 2 and 3, naming and describing a variety of human capacities, are all important to ethics. Neurobiologist Donald Pfaff asserts that "the brain does not have a signaling system dedicated to ethics."[6] Nor, we might add, does it have a signaling system dedicated to religion, chess moves, cooking a soufflé, playing the cello, or watching Monday Night Football. But we hardly need a neuroscientist to tell us this. Even a moment's reflection shows that moral experiences are different in the head and in the gut, different still in the imagination, when placed into narrative form, or enacted in a ritual. And each of these, in various situations, may turn out to be the right form for appreciating a moral experience and solving an ethical problem. The heart, mind, memory, imagination, various bodily gestures, and many other faculties and capacities can be in play, and it would be presumptive to say in advance which is likely to be most helpful. It stands to reason that if there are different kinds of moral experiences, then different human faculties will be involved. If there is no master faculty, no Supreme Court of the moral life, then we are wise to resist the idea that there is some best way to reach resolution or that even reaching resolution will be a recognizable and more-or-less standard event. In short, moral pluralism is thoroughgoing, reaching all the way through our embodied selves.

One compelling piece of evidence for this depth is that so many different ethical texts stretching over thousands of years continue to have resonance. Otherwise, students of ethics wouldn't still be reading Aristotle, Epictetus, Augustine, and Aquinas, as well as Martin Luther King, John Rawls, Martha Nussbaum, Carol Gilligan, and many others—each of whom appeals to different capacities and different scenarios in the human moral dynamic as they offer their theories (and antitheories), methods, and processes. And one can detect this variation by noting the kinds of illustrations and examples each of these writers assumes as the basic problem set that engages our ethical capacities.

Because of this complexity in the human moral dynamic, it becomes very important to listen carefully to the language people are using when they are grappling with moral issues, listening not just for their insights, but for the processes and methods they use to reach them and the way they are held or embedded within a person's moral biography. And if this sort of listening is important for our dealings with others, it is also important for our own moral self-understanding.

As noted in chapter 3, listening to ourselves—to our inner and outer moral dialogues—is an essential skill of ethics, as it leads to what I call there an "assertive skill," the recognition and claiming of our own moral authority. Careful listening will help me distinguish among those inner voices vying for supremacy, such as my father's voice; the voices of consumerism, tribalism, or influential friends; or the seductive voice of my ego. I am not arguing that there is one, true, distinctive voice for each individual that must be discovered among the cacophonous multitude, but simply for the need to choose, and assume responsibility for, the voice I choose among the many contenders. Listening for, choosing, and affirming my own voice in ethics help me appreciate that the same task, and a similar complexity, is also at work in others.

Moral judgments are not free-standing but nested in complex patterns of meaning. My work not only with students but also with patients, families, and clinicians in the context of decisions about medical care is my most consistent window into the great pluralism of moral norms, processes, methods, and languages. Forgoing our desire for a final or unifying definition of ethics is an important move in the ongoing effort to honor this pluralism and understand its role in our lives.

The idea that there is some special human faculty, some moral sense, that serves as a final judge is a staple of Western moral philosophy and a conviction frequently encountered in contemporary society. Recently I made the claim to a group of lawyers that there was no such single human faculty. There was serious objection from the audience that I had not sufficiently considered conscience. Conscience *can* work in this way as the final adjudicator of right and wrong, but only if we could insulate the workings of conscience from the influence of personal histories (including prehistories), cultural context, and the traditional beliefs and practices of communities. Still, we might follow the lead of Joseph Butler, who makes conscience something like a divine implant, to be trusted because of its superhuman origins.[7] But, on examination, this divinely inspired faculty quickly begins to look worrisome, even to theists, since people identify its contents and signaling system very differently. I refer the reader to the section on conscience in chapter 7.

Restricting What Experiences Have Ethical Weight

During the early years of the twenty-first century several medical institutions were involved in testing a new and promising treatment for spina bifida. In babies with spina bifida, a portion of the neural tube fails to develop properly in utero, leaving an opening in the back and causing defects in the spinal cord and the bones of the spine. The problems resulting from spina bifida can range from mild to severe, depending on the type of defect and its size, location, and complications. The treatment under investigation involved a complex process of opening the uterus, removing the fetus for surgery to close the back, and returning the fetus to the uterus for continued gestation. The aim was to reduce newborn hydrocephaly (excess fluid in the brain, causing swelling and neurological damage), potential paralysis, and developmental delays. Infants with hydrocephaly require shunts to drain off the excess cerebral fluid. Shunts can become infected or clogged, and the additional surgeries required to repair or replace them are thought to be a major insult to the infant brain, reducing intellectual potential and exacerbating physical disabilities.

While fetal surgery for lethal conditions is a well-established practice, spina bifida—while resulting in significant handicaps—is a nonlethal condition. The controversy arises because fetal surgery for spina bifida involves a small risk of mortality to both the fetus and the mother. Because it was at that time an experimental procedure, the local Institutional Review Board (an ethical review body for research involving human subjects) required that a rigorous informed consent process be provided to the parents prior to embarking on the surgery. I was involved as an informed consent monitor for one of these trials. In this role I interviewed the parents to try to ascertain whether they had an adequate understanding of the risks and benefits of the experimental surgery, that is, enough of an understanding that their consent or refusal to participate was informed. As such, I was privy to the reasoning of the parents about this surgery and the moral judgment concerning whether to undergo it. One of the most striking features of what I learned was the importance of unanticipated elements in the parents' decisions.

In decision-making, people are in search of moral coherence and integrity in their lives, and in this search for coherence and integrity, unexpected features can play an important part. One young woman I interviewed gave the following account of her decision to undergo the surgery.

> This may sound weird to you, but since my grandfather passed away, I've felt this presence like he was watching over me and my baby. And in my heart and mind I feel like he's going to be watching over us if I have this procedure done. He's not going to let anything [bad] happen.

(I describe this interview in greater detail in the section on spirituality in chapter 6. Readers should also know that this young woman missed her grandfather's funeral to keep her appointment at the medical center to learn about fetal surgery.)

Another woman reflected on the way her decision was grounded in her religious beliefs and indicated how something that would have otherwise been insignificant signaled to her on this occasion that the right path was to proceed to the surgery.

> I am a Christian, and I believe in the Bible. That's just who we are. Last Friday when I found out about the spina bifida I was having all these horrible visions . . . you know, how life from here on is going to be horrible. And we [she and her husband] were debating this. Then I went to my mailbox and pulled out a magazine—it's called *Decision Magazine* [a publication of the Billy Graham Evangelistic Association], and it says on the cover, "Your strength in the storm," and this is our faith. And when I got that I said "Whew. OK, All right. My faith—this is why I have faith, for these kinds of situations."

She and her husband subsequently chose the experimental fetal surgery.

Yet another couple was thrust into a deeply reflective mode when they discovered that the hotel in which they were staying near the medical center was located on Mt. Moriah Church Road. This connected in their sensibility to the story in Genesis and to the site, Mount Moriah, on which Abraham was commanded to sacrifice his son Isaac, only to be reprieved at the last minute, as Abraham spotted a ram in the bushes to take the place of Isaac.

Questions about responsibilities to children, born and unborn, figured heavily into the decisions of all the couples I interviewed. Yet likely no one would have anticipated that the pivot points for these decisions lay where they did—in the felt protective presence of a deceased grandfather, in the receipt of a magazine in the mail, or in the discovery of a street name symbolic of faith in a divine pardon for one's child. My point here is that elements that might have been unimaginable at the beginning of a decision process proved to be major pivot points.

Restricting the kinds of human experiences that can carry ethical weight is always a mistake. There is no remedy for this pitfall except careful probing, attentive listening, and especially stretching one's imagination to encompass a very wide range of experiences as morally instructive. Some readers may be reluctant to accredit these personal interpretations of what is morally significant and view them as irrational. Yet to do so would be to miss the powerful dynamics that give ethical choices their coherence and ordering power in our lives. Willingness to embrace novel features during decision-making is one way to honor the wide expanse of moral experiences and the interpretive generosity of the human mind.

Treating Mysteries as Moral Problems

Not everything that puzzles us is a moral problem. The twentieth-century French existentialist Gabriel Marcel distinguishes between *problems* and *mysteries*.[8] Problem have solutions; moral problems have better and worse ways of being resolved. The skills and capacities I emphasize in this volume have purchase on these problems and can yield results. Mysteries, by contrast, do not have solutions, and the appropriate demeanor toward them is living with them and respecting the ways they exceed our capacities for understanding. Mysteries put us in our place. They require a bit of humility and sometimes reverence.

Whether to arm teachers to reduce mass killings in schools is a question with social, political, and ethical aspects. It can be answered based on evidence, what sort of role teachers have, and what role they should have. It is in part empirical, in part cultural, and in part ethical. It is complex because it concerns us both as individuals and as communities. But, despite its complexity, it is amenable to an answer. We may have to work hard to grasp its long-range implications, but it is not beyond us. It may challenge us morally and intellectually, but calm, deliberate, and imaginative thinking are the appropriate tools for responding.

By contrast, the moral issues surrounding abortion contain a profound mystery. When during gestation is a human life present, that is, a human life that has the same dignity and rights that we attribute to ourselves? Of course, there are a variety of ways that an answer has been attempted. The official Roman Catholic position is that human life, of equal value to the mother's, begins at the moment of conception. This is essentially an argument based on theological doctrine and genetic uniqueness and ignores developmental differences between a one-day-old conceptus and a full-term fetus. Other ways of positing the presence of a full, rights-bearing human being, a person, draw the line at some point in fetal development, for example, at viability, following the 1973 U.S. Supreme Court ruling in *Roe v. Wade*. Others assign personhood when there is a detectable heartbeat, or a primitive brain, as indicated by the presence of the neural tube. Yet every effort to establish definitively the presence of a person within unborn life involves many suppositions and leaps of reason, emphasizing some features while neglecting others, so that the answers always contain a level of arbitrariness. The question is best described not as a problem to be solved, but as a mystery to be lived with. When human life begins is not an empirical question, since there is no definitive set of evidentiary tests that are compelling. Nor is it an ethical question, such that with the exercise of the skills we have discussed and sustained moral analysis, an answer will become evident. The emergence of personhood is a question before which we should be agnostic and, therefore, humble. It is a mystery, and all efforts to answer it in some definitive way to shore up an ethical position should be rejected.

This does not mean, to be sure, that there are no moral dimensions to reproduction and termination; it does not mean that rules about better and worse actions and laws with boundaries are impossible to devise. It simply means that whatever moral judgments and social policies we adopt are efforts to muddle through. Good ethics and good laws about abortion have no greater status than "the best we can do for now," given how little we really know and the ineptness of our tools. Mysteries, unlike problems, do not admit to greater transparency through more careful thinking. They remain opaque, and our rules, policies, and laws are no more than efforts to make sense of how to live with this mystery.

Respecting the mystery in defining personhood helps us respect the mysterious within us, including the mystery we are to ourselves. There are also mysterious elements in close relationships—dimensions that defy definition or complete analysis. These qualities are common in long friendships and in marriages and intimate partnerships, where the ineffable features of the bond between people inspire something like awe and reverence. Katherine Anne Porter has described this well. Marriage, she says, is an estate publicly affirmed but symbolic of a deeper, secret, and mystical alliance—"mystical exactly in the sense that the real experience cannot be communicated to others, nor explained even to oneself on rational grounds."[9]

In brief, mystery has an important place in ethics, not as part of a problem-solving strategy but as a discernment that marks the boundary beyond which ethical analysis cannot go. The acknowledgment that some things we encounter are ineffable and unanalyzable realities should evoke in us attitudes of wonderment, awe, and reverence. Recognizing this reality is one of the chief shields against hubris.

6
Moral Concepts in Practice I

What moral concepts are central to a good life? I have selected 11 to examine in this chapter and the one that follows. A comprehensive treatment of these ideas is not possible in a short book, and my intention is less to speak about them definitively and more to signal their important uses. Each concept does essential moral work, and each has a place in a well-formed moral sensibility, although each also has limitations and misuses. Some of the concepts I have selected are ones that might be found in any ethics text, such as "truth," "responsibility," "liberty," "rights," "justice," and "conscience." Others are relatively neglected in contemporary ethics scholarship but are inevitable components of a reflective life. In this category are "forgiveness," "love," "spirituality," "hope," and "death." In exploring the meanings and uses of these concepts I occasionally rely on novelists, poets, and religious thinkers. The interplay of life experiences with these concepts is often captured more powerfully in literature than in philosophical analysis.

I also have a lifespan approach in mind. Moral ideas that have little relevance at one point in our life journey often become critically important concepts at a later stage. Death is a good example; it may have little meaning for us in our youth but become axial as we lose people we love or face our own mortality. Love and spirituality also have shifting valences depending on where we are in the lifespan. Forgiveness usually increases in importance the older we are, simply because there have been more opportunities for mistakes. The importance of truth is constant, but the need for it increases when it loses favor socially and politically, as in the present.

In chapters 2 and 3, I describe some basic skills needed for ethics. If ethical thinking were formulaic, we could expect to match skills with these concepts in some precise way. For example, it would be tempting to think that an understanding of love will primarily involve emotional skill. Yet working with love as a moral concept requires a variety of skills, for example, emotional, cognitive, and imaginative. Our life experiences and our situation will determine which skills are needed to work with which concepts.

The Anchoring Value of Truth

Why is truth-telling such an important fixture for ethics? We all lie and do so routinely. Let us say, for example, that my favorite aunt gives me a tie for my birthday that is not just a bad color but of garish design. I wouldn't wear it to a dogfight. She is obviously solicitous of my approval. Do I say, "I would have to be in my coffin to be dressed in this thing" or find some way to save her feelings? The latter course will involve lying, here meaning finding some way to deceive her and spare her embarrassment. I might say, "Thank you so much for remembering my birthday." Whether this would do the trick or more embellishment and enthusiasm are needed, of course, depends a lot on just who this aunt is and our interactions in the past. But the point here is that we often lie to people to spare their feelings, shield them from embarrassment, or prevent awkwardness. The truth, and a demeanor of truthfulness on our part, is not the highest principle of ethics in all situations. And describing the full context of lying should be enough to make the case that deviating from the truth, if not the absolute right thing, is at least sometimes an acceptable moral option.

So, if lying is common, why it is almost universally viewed as a problem? A transition in medical norms and practices in the recent past may help to answer this question. For decades ethicists have debated the moral appropriateness of doctors lying to their patients. Traditions of paternalistic benevolence are long and deep in the history of medical ethics. An obligation of truthfulness to patients did not explicitly enter the Code of Ethics of the American Medical Association until 1980. Social and medical norms have changed dramatically since that time, and now lying to patients, especially those who are severely ill or dying, is typically frowned upon, even when families request it. Still, it is instructive to look at the usual reasons given for lying to patients as a register for why we are tempted to lie generally, since the reasons given are typically associated with an underlying moral disregard for persons.

Physicians and their apologists have argued as follows.

- The truth can be harmful to patients and increase their suffering. In situations of incurable illnesses, the truth is cruel and contrary to obligations to maintain a patient's hope.
- Patients are incapable of understanding the truth. They don't have medical degrees and misunderstand probabilities of success and failure associated with therapeutic options. Doctors are trained to understand these decisions and thereby have an obligation to make them.
- Patients do not want to know the truth. Already compromised by their illnesses, patients recognize they are in a dependence relationship and want doctors to protect them from the burden of decisions.

The obligation to truthfulness *is* always contextual, but this doesn't mean it is relative. Telling the truth must be the default position, and exceptions to it need to be justified by appeal to exceptional circumstances. As Sissela Bok puts it, "lying requires a *reason*, while truth-telling does not."[1] The previously discussed rationales show how temptations to lie often disclose other moral problems. Take the first one. It is a thin and superficial view of persons that assumes they will lose hope if given a discouraging diagnosis (see discussion under "The Persistence of Hope" later in this chapter). It infantilizes patients rather than accrediting them with strength, character, and personal resources. Most of us have been through at least some hard times before we hear a severe or terminal diagnosis, and depriving us of the information dramatically underestimates the moral and spiritual resources we possess. The second rationale, that patients can't understand, infantilizes patients in another way—through assumptions of both ignorance and lesser cognitive capacities. No patient is ever likely to understand as much as a medical professional does about the details of a diagnosis and prognosis, but most of us can understand enough to discern whether the disease we have is serious and the pros and cons of whatever options may be available. The third rationale, that patients don't want to know, is perhaps the worst, since it imputes dubious motives and intentions to patients. This third rationale is the most directly paternalistic, although each arrives at this destination. Beneficent paternalism is usually a cover for the health professional who is too uncomfortable to be candid or feels inept at relating to patients when there is a diminished possibility of helping them. Sadly, the cases of patient abandonment I have witnessed were grounded in precisely this ineptness and fear. All three strategies for dealing with difficult information belittle patients and cut them off from the kind of human contact that people with severe diagnoses need the most.

Physicians are no different from the rest of us. We all tend to cloak our deceptions in a variety of good intentions, a superordinate beneficence that submerges the other person's distinctive self. I do not argue that lying is never morally acceptable, and I have tried to make the case in the previous discussion that on rare occasions it is praiseworthy. But lying has become so routine in public life that its corrosive effect is apparent everywhere; it has become more the rule than the exception that proves the rule. It belittles and stigmatizes; in public life it usually has nothing to do with beneficent intentions and is most often a cloak for rampant self-interest. Almost all lies undermine trust that is essential for a functioning society, not to mention a working friendship or stable family life. If we cannot rely on each other to tell the truth, we have nothing to build on.

Imagine a situation in which I have routinely and habitually lied about how I am using a pool of funds that you and I agree are only for our common purposes. I use these funds for my own ends and then lie to you periodically about where the money has gone. This goes on for months, and when the money is finally all expended on my pet projects, bad investments, gambling debts, or drug use, I realize I must come clean. Now I insist I am telling you the truth. But by this time my credibility is gone. I can say, "I lied before, but I really am telling you the truth now!" My past pattern of lying leaves grave doubts in your mind, and whatever assumptions of probity we began with are now long gone. To the habitual or chronic liar, we are always justified in asking, "Why should I believe you now or any time in the future?" Once the standard is eroded it takes a great deal to reestablish it. In marriages and friendships, it is exceedingly difficult. In job performance and for elected officials, such trust may never be re-established.

One reason to be skeptical about the future veracity of persons who lie, beyond the loss of trust, is that habitual or persistent lying has a corrosive effect on the liar. One lie often requires another to cover the original deception and establishes a pattern. It is just such patterns and habits that form character. Again, Sissela Bok has an apt phrase: "It is easy . . . to tell a lie, but hard to tell only one."[2] We recognize this from our own efforts to cover our deceptions.

Disregard for the truth jeopardizes many of the core assumptions we make about how relationships work, and in this sense, truth is a foundation stone for both personal and social cohesiveness. A society that no longer assumes that truth is essential for its core interactions devolves into a corrosive cynicism and ripens the culture for just the sort of moral egoism that Thomas Hobbes describes in *Leviathan*. Yet we may have already entered a period of "post-truth."

The staff of Oxford Dictionaries chose "post-truth" as its "word of the year" in 2016.[3] This term means "relating to or denoting circumstances in which objective facts are less influential in shaping public opinion than appeals to emotion and personal belief."[3] It is clear we are in a post-truth political era. Counterfactual claims are repeated in seemingly endless tweets, videos, and even newscasts. Emotional appeals unconnected to facts dominate as accurate details about decisions and policies are ignored.

One distressing dimension of a post-truth political culture is the frequency of ad hominem arguments, literally, arguments "to the person." An ad hominem argument is one that attacks the person making the argument rather than the argument itself. It focuses on some feature, attribute, or interest of the person as disqualifying him or her from having a valid viewpoint on the issue at hand. Here's an example: "Karl Marx couldn't be right in his economic theories. He couldn't even consistently feed his own family." Ad hominem assertions are sometimes made to completely disqualify entire categories or groups of persons from participating in moral debates. For example, the views of atheists are often attacked and discounted under the suggestion or implication that they have lax moral standards and cannot be trusted with matters of the public good.

Ad hominem arguments are considered fallacies of reasoning. Their appeal is completely emotional and prejudicial. They are effective because falling back on our preconceptions and prejudices is often easier than stopping to think or rethink our position. We have a natural tendency to think the worst of those who disagree with us, or at least fail to give them the benefit of the doubt. Thus, we are all subject to the prejudicial temptations of ad hominem suggestions and gestures, even when they are not explicitly or completely expressed.

Yet the problem of ad hominem assertions is not just that they play on prejudice and villainize those who disagree with us. This problem is compounded by the tendency in such assertions to embellish, fabricate, or plainly lie. This progression is easy to understand. If character assassination is the aim, a moral line has already been crossed. The opponent is already less than human and so piling on a few more assertions of dubious validity, or simply lying, seems not so much a new boundary crossed as a natural extension of the original aim to discredit.

When truth is disregarded as a moral standard, disregard for the dignity of persons will follow.

Forgiveness and Freedom

How can we repair relationships after a moral breach? How do we keep moral mistakes, violations, and betrayals from becoming enduring fissures that damage our lives and those around us? This question is rarely taken up in philosophical discourse, but it is customary fare for most religious traditions. Yet regardless of one's religious convictions, or lack thereof, forgiveness does important ethical work.

Forgiveness is an activity of moral well-being. If we are unable or unwilling to forgive transgressions against us, we tend to create a moral identity around our injuries. We keep score and overidentify around the slights and insults that we all from time to time receive, so that we hang on to, even nurture and prize, our injuries. If I do this scorekeeping, I largely reduce my moral biography to victimization. I create a narrative that revolves around, perhaps even embellishes, these insults and the pain they cause, and this becomes the story of my life.

An extreme case of this self-absorption in nursing one's injury is Miss Havisham of Charles Dickens's *Great Expectations*.[4] Left at the altar on her wedding day by a suitor who robbed her of her fortune, she continued to wear her wedding dress the rest of her life, stopped all clocks at the time she first learned of the betrayal, and left the wedding feast rotting on the dining table for the rats and mice. In typical Dickensian fashion, Miss Havisham's subsequent actions result in inadvertent injury to others whom she loves. Forgiveness becomes a part of the story, but only near her death. The larger moral of the story is how motivation, intention, and judgment become warped and even perverse because of living a life story centered on an injury one does not move beyond.

The negative baggage from holding on to hurts leads to a truncated, diminished sense of moral selfhood. The work of forgiveness is what has enabled us to tell different stories about our identities and thus create renewed moral selves. So, the benefits of forgiveness are not just reconciling us to estranged others but creating a self with a more open future.

This work of forgiveness has been highlighted by the political philosopher Hannah Arendt in her classic work *The Human Condition*.[5] Arendt begins with a recognition that human actions often have unpredictable and irreversible effects for both ourselves and others. She does not concern herself with willed evil or malicious actions, but with the way that every human activity has a power to disrupt and damage despite lack of malice.

Arendt's view is that people need to forgive to move beyond these breaches, to allow them to begin anew, and not forever be tied to the trail of consequences stemming from such transgressions. "Trespassing is an everyday occurrence," she says, "which is in the very nature of action's constant establishment of new relationships within a web of relations, and it needs forgiving, dismissing, in order to make it possible for life to go on."[6] Forgiveness is a kind of releasing that is necessary for people to remain free agents, to act again, and be trusted once more in their actions.

For Arendt, the chief contrast with forgiveness is vengeance. Vengeance means reacting in kind to the original wronging activity. Forgiveness stops the revenge cycle of an eye for an eye and allows relationships to begin anew. It is "freedom from vengeance, which encloses both doer and sufferer."[7]

Injuries can be the minor insults of daily life or more serious and damaging injuries—some intentional; others, accidents or mishaps. They may involve no malice but result from the routine lapses of ordinary life: a careless offensive remark that hurts a friend's feelings, postponed car maintenance results in an accident that injures a bystander, or a severed nerve in a surgical complication that is a known risk discussed in the informed consent process.

Some injuries are so large, however, that we think of them as crimes, and we may wonder whether they are beyond forgiveness. In *The Sunflower*, Simon Wiesenthal presents the story of a young Jew listening silently as a dying Nazi begs absolution for taking part in the burning alive of an entire village of Jews.[8] A range of commentaries follow this story, but the intent of the book as a whole is to leave the reader with the query of whether forgiveness is even possible here. While forgiveness may or may not be feasible, it is not a substitute for justice nor for rectifying—to the extent possible—the rips in the social fabric from such crimes.

One of the most interesting possibilities to consider ethically is whether one can or should forgive an injury in the absence of an apology or, in more serious injuries, in the absence of efforts to make restitution. This question may arise for several reasons. Sometimes the person who has injured me has died. In some situations, the injury is remote in time and has been forgotten by the person who caused it. In other cases the injuring party refuses to see that any harm has been done. If the stakes for the moral self are high, as I have argued, then forgiveness may be important in all these circumstances. I may simply not want my life shaped by the transgression and need to move beyond both the injury and the offending party. Forgiving in these circumstances, as in others, is a move to a less encumbered future. Finding a way to forgive oneself and others is a path to freedom.

The Varieties of Love

Many important concepts fly under the banner of "love," each with its own moral significance. Until very recently, Anglo-American philosophers have largely overlooked love as a moral concept. Martha Nussbaum is a notable exception, and she argues that the reason for this dearth of attention is because Western ethics is so focused on choices and acts of will.[9] Love, by contrast, is usually seen as involuntary, something one "falls" into, is subjected to, or is overcome by. Feminist philosophers have been the most persistent in the effort to make at least one aspect of love, caring, a prominent part of morals, and their efforts should lead us to question both the idea that ethics is always about voluntary choices and that the affections are always involuntary. As argued in chapter 2, we have choices about how to understand and relate to our emotional states—which to act upon, which to ignore, and which to refine and expand as valuable parts of ourselves.

Assessments of love in theological ethics are typically more lucid about its importance, yet religious teachings usually couch their inquiries into love within larger theological aims. Consequently, these teachings often explore love by contrasting two modes, namely, contrasting the love of God with all other—and presumably inferior—forms of love. This framing limits its usefulness as a core moral term needed to describe a great range of human affections and attachments.

Religious practices expressing and embodying love are far richer sources for moral understanding than theological doctrine. Just as moral acts are more complex than the moral concepts that try to describe and explain them, religious rituals and practices typically outstrip in meaning and depth the theology they supposedly reflect. While I will not take up the task here, those who want to understand the depth and sophistication of religious understandings of love would do better to observe what religious people do rather than read the doctrines and pronouncements of religious leaders.

Etymology helpfully illustrates the broad range of concepts of love. There are at least four Greek terms that can be translated as love.

- Eros—passionate, physical love, longing and desire; "falling in love"
- Philia—love between friends, in Aristotle the high-minded affection of people who recognize something valuable in each other
- Agape—spiritually inspired, sacrificial love; the term used in the Christian Gospels for the love of God
- Storge—the affection that emerges from the mutual care of daily life, as in a family; not "falling in love" but "living in a place of love."

One of the striking things in considering this short list is how many kinds of affection and how many human relationships these terms cover. Each form has particular moral aspects and implications and is just a beginning catalogue for the many circumstances in which love plays a pivotal role. Consider the following: the love of parents for children and siblings for each other; the love of spouses and long-term partners for each other; the love of a professor for her students and the reciprocal (sometimes) affection of students for those who have diligently tried to educate them; the affection of colleagues who work together for long periods on an arduous assignment; the love between clinicians and their patients; the love of soldiers in battle for each other; the love of country; the love of work; the love of ideas; the love of baseball; the love of music; the love for a pet; the love for a great piece of literature or art. A local artist sitting in my den, in which one of her early works was hanging, spontaneously turned to the painting and said to it, with as sincere an intonation as I have ever heard, "I love you!"

Not all movements of the affections are best described as love, but many of them are. A plaque in Westminster Abbey honoring novelist George Eliot (Mary Ann Evans) captures the centrality of love for the moral life: "The first condition of human goodness is something to love; the second something to reverence." Humans need something outside themselves to give their affections to be morally whole. In part, this describes the deep need we have for social relationships, for bonds of affection with others. Love directed solely to the self turns toxic or, as described in chapter 2 in the fable of Narcissus, deadly. In terms of understanding how ethics works, Eliot's observation also implies that an ethical preoccupation with duties and responsibilities is dramatically limited and stultifying. I need moral exemplars who will not only teach me my duty, but also show me how to love, how to respect, nurture, and direct my affections. Perhaps more than anything else, finding the right things to love, in the right way, is the crucial step in finding human fulfillment.

A distinctive contribution to the moral importance of love in the twentieth and twenty-first centuries has been made by female and feminist writers. I focus on three representative thinkers who have a special interest in the ethics of care: Sara Ruddick, Virginia Held, and Eva Kittay. Each is indebted to the pioneering work of Carol Gilligan, discussed in chapter 5 in the section "Expecting Too Much from Theory."

Sara Ruddick's 1989 book, *Maternal Thinking*, describes the importance and need for public recognition of mothering as a central moral practice, including preserving, nurturing, and fostering the growth of children into adulthood.[10] In *The Ethics of Care*, Virginia Held also endorses a maternal paradigm and stresses the shortcoming of the male model that assumes that an ethics covering issues of competition, negotiating conflict, and disinterested fairness is adequate.[11] She argues for greater balance in which norms of cooperation, consensus, and community are equally important. The male model is not wrong, she asserts, but rather a moral minimum. A robust ethics of caring, as in healthy families and well-functioning friendships, is necessary for anything like a full human life. Kittay's work, such as *Love's Labor*, argues for a recognition of the work of caretaking and the need to empower workers who take care of the dependency needs of others.[12]

These authors are important for my purposes because by centering their work on caring practices they broaden and deepen our understanding of this form of love as an axis around which moral life turns. Their work is a sobering reminder that the dominant operating portrait of persons making independent moral judgments is deeply flawed. Even our most seemingly independent actions are preceded and followed by dependence on others who support and nurture us. The life cycle runs from a radical dependence in infancy and childhood, to relative independence in adulthood, to a return to dependence in old age. This rhythm of interdependence should inform and shape our ethical paradigm. And this paradigm is unintelligible without various forms of love threaded through it at all stages. Walt Whitman says it best in *Leaves of Grass*: "A kelson of the creation is love."[13] In other words, just as a kelson is the structural line that holds a ship together, love—in various forms—is the integral element that holds a life together.

The Buddhist metta prayer also carries this implication of love as a great integral, binding force, which we have an obligation to will and project across time and space. It begins with directing loving kindness toward oneself in words such as "May I love myself, be blessed and happy," extending this intention in an ever-widening circle to others who are near, such as family and neighbors, and then to those who are more distant, and also to enemies, and finally to all beings: "May all beings everywhere, whether near or far, whether known to me or unknown, be loved and happy. May they be well. May they be peaceful. May they be free."

The Moral Uses of Spirituality

What is spirituality, and how does it function in ethics? I begin with a practical definition of spirituality and then describe how spiritual values are connected to and translated into ethical practices.

Several years ago, I was talking with a young, expectant mother whose fetus had been diagnosed with spina bifida, incomplete closure of the fetal spine with accompanying problems of paralysis and mental development. (I describe other facets of this conversation in chapter 5, under "Restricting What Experiences Have Ethical Weight.") She was being offered participation in a research protocol designed to lessen the developmental problems associated with spina bifida through prenatal surgery. I was functioning as a consent monitor, trying to ensure that she and other subjects who entered this surgical trial understood what they were getting into. This young woman insisted that she wasn't worried about any of the risks of the surgery. She said she felt the presence of God, mediated through her recently deceased grandfather, and that he had not warned her away from this procedure, so she knew the surgery would go well. "Oh," I said, "is religion then a big part of your decision about whether to have this procedure?" To which she replied, "No." Religion to her meant churches, ministers, and the metaphysical furniture of Christianity, which had little meaning for her, but she felt and trusted the presence of God. By her own reckoning, she was a spiritual, but not a religious, person. My assumptions were too restrictive; I was thinking about spiritual matters from within a box labeled "religion." What this young woman embodied was an innate human capacity for seeking and finding transcendent meaning at critical junctures in life.

    The basis for understanding contemporary thinking about spirituality and religion begins in the late nineteenth and early twentieth centuries with scholars like William James and Rudolf Otto—and later Joachim Wach and Mircea Eliade—who sought to understand religion as a *human* phenomenon. They meant that religious experience is simply a natural human capacity, a distinctive kind of experience that can be studied and appreciated without being tied to doctrinal teachings or metaphysical trappings. Theology, they said, is too often in the service of institutional agendas, constricted to stating the truth about God from within a tradition of faith and practice. The study of religion as a human phenomenon, by contrast, brackets the question of truth to perceive, explore, and describe.

Accordingly, these scholars invented new terminology. Rudolf Otto, for example, used the term "numinous" to refer to the sense of holiness, mystery, and awe that religious experiences evoke.[14] Mircea Eliade, in his extensive comparative cataloguing of religious experiences in the East and West, talked about "the sacred."[15] Wach characterizes religious experience as a response of awe to what is perceived as ultimate reality.[16] This way of thinking is now widely recognized and practiced, primarily because of its appreciative embrace of pluralism. It opens religious experiences universally to humankind, and it situates them within ordinary, human capabilities. William James said it definitively more than a century ago in his Gifford Lectures at the University of Edinburgh when he claimed that his approach democratizes the religious impulse.[17] It releases religion from being the property of particular communities, like churches, or special people, like priests or "believers," or even academic scholars of religion. It also frees religion from exclusive identification with specific human capacities, like "believing," or specific religious doctrines, like "belief in a supreme creator." In other words, from James's perspective, it is characteristic of religion that everyone is capable of it, that every time, place, and event is a potential vehicle for religious meaning, and every human faculty a potential conduit for religious insight.

This noninstitutionalized form of religion is what many Americans now refer to as "spirituality." I am using the term in this inclusive sense, which can include the usual institutional forms of religion but goes beyond them. What scholars of religion discovered is that there will inevitably be a great variety of religious experiences and forms of expression—a plurality of religious truth and meaning. It is characteristic of this new understanding that there are no predetermined limits to what can be a vehicle for the sacred or the kinds of human activity that can be conduits to a transcendent understanding. The psychologist Abraham Maslow called these "peak-experiences," and his research suggested they were common to our species.[18] In these highly focused and concentrated peaks, the universe is perceived as a sublimely beautiful, integrated whole, with a superordinate reality and worth, in which ordinary ego concerns fall away. Sometimes this happens for people when they are hiking in Yellowstone or holding a newborn child or grandchild. But it can be something as simple as waking up on a Tuesday morning with the certain knowledge that every rock and tree, every clump of dirt and blade of grass, is sacred. Perhaps this broad and inclusive understanding of spirituality is especially appealing to Americans. It was Walt Whitman, after all, who said that he sees God in every hour, every human face, including his own, and finds "letters from God dropped in the street, and every one is signed by God's name."[19]

Philosophical discussions of the place and role of spiritual insights for ethics are often confined to consideration of what is called "divine command theory." In brief, this theory says that actions are good or right because they are commanded by God, who is perceived as the ultimate authority and sole instructor for moral values. A compelling counterargument to this theory dates at least as far back as the Platonic dialogue *Euthyphro*. The essence of the counterargument is that there must a separate standard for moral values, that is, something more than the fact that it is commanded by God. If divine commands are all that we have to justify actions, then we would be obligated to kill nonbelievers if God commanded us to do so. In other words, divine command theory makes ethics arbitrary. It also makes all the tools and capacities of human moral judgment inoperable. Using the example of a divine command to kill others makes it clear that, despite its flaws, this perspective is alive and well, operative in the minds of many religious fundamentalists, including those who wage terror. When divine commands are perceived to be operative in a culture, they must be subjected to the same critical scrutiny given to all moral claims to authority, regardless of the source.

Yet the significance of spirituality for ethics is far greater than the arguments and counterarguments for divine command theory. A great many spiritual and religious people ground their moral activity in their sense of the sacred. The section in chapter 5 entitled "Restricting What Experiences Have Ethical Weight" provides three examples of the complex workings of spirituality in ethical decision-making. Indeed, the high stakes and uncertainties that mark many ethical decisions make them fertile ground for perceptions and discernments that are spiritual in nature. Following Maslow's research, we know that peak experiences are powerful in a way that ordinary experiences are not, and part of that power lies in a conviction that what is revealed through them is more "real" than what happens in daily life. Thus, the content of spiritual insights—such as oneness with the universe, the supremacy of goodness, a sense of deep belonging, and a self empty of ego—becomes the template against which ethical life is measured. Working with such a template requires virtues such as patience, imagination, respect for others, courage, and perseverance, as well as kindness and other forms of love. The best uses of spiritual insights are those that help us locate and act upon some of our most cherished moral norms.

The Persistence of Hope

Hope is morally important because it enables some essential virtues, such as courage, perseverance, patience, and openness to the future. Aristotle, for example, linked hope with courage in his discussion of cowardice: "The coward, then, is a despairing sort of person; for he fears everything. The brave man, on the other hand, has the opposite disposition; for confidence is the mark of a hopeful disposition."[20] In this sense, hope or, more precisely, hopefulness is of deep ethical importance as an empowering capacity. Hopeful people can simply do things that those without hope cannot, thus enabling a fruition and flourishing of human potential. As philosopher Judith Andre puts it, "lack of hope undercuts most worldly virtues."[21]

Initially, it is important to distinguish hope from optimism, a weak and flawed alternative. Terry Eagleton describes optimism as the U.S. "state ideology"—an unremitting positivity and compulsive cheeriness.[22] The optimist feels compelled at every turn to say, "Life will be good," while harboring a fear that it won't be, thus magnifying the seductiveness of magical thinking. Optimism is often a thin veil for cloaking unwanted realities, and in this deceptive covering of life's harshness, it makes courage, perseverance, patience, and openness to truth unnecessary.

By contrast, hope is always a demeanor adopted after encountering and reflectively taking in life's bruises and disappointments. Hope relies on realism for its power. It has its greatest usefulness in difficult times, when it would be easy to give up. In this sense, the opposite of hope is despair. Andre argues that one of the advantages of hope over a facile optimism is that being hopeful releases all the energy absorbed in optimism's resistance and denial.[23] And unlike optimism, hope is not subject to utopian entrapment.

Twentieth-century existentialist Gabriel Marcel makes a distinction between "I hope . . . ," the categorical affirmation, and "I hope that . . . ," that is, hoping for specific outcomes. For Marcel, the ontological gesture "I hope" is how the temptation to despair at the ills and evils of the world is overcome.[24] As a virtue, hope is not an attitude but a practice, gradually learned and refined in a community and, in the best societies, in a civil polity that seeks to promote solidarity and bring out the best in people. Hope, then, differs from even the best forms of optimism because it is not a function of temperament but is a learned practice in the face of difficulty.

Hope is an important virtue for clinicians and counselors and for all of us who are placed in roles of advising, whether professionally or personally. One informal rule I heard repeatedly in medical circles was that a clinician should never take away a patient's hope. This is sometimes a rationale for deception around a terminal diagnosis, sometimes a rationale for offering the patient experimental procedures of little promise and substantial risk, and sometimes a rationale for failing to give specifics in a diagnosis. Each of these strategies runs a very serious risk that patients will fail to understand just how seriously ill they are. I think these dubious actions are based on an underestimate of people's resilience in the face of bad news and on a failure to understand how hope works, as previously depicted. Hope as a demeanor of one's life is not the sort of thing that can be easily undermined, so it is not the sort of thing that a clinician, even one who enjoys the patient's trust, can easily "take away." Unlike optimism, hard times are occasions when hope shines. In Greek mythology, the box Pandora opened releasing all the ills for humankind also contained the spirit of hope.

Part of the problem in the previously depicted clinician–patient scenario is the faulty assumption that we can predict what people hope for; it is not always survival. Those with terminal diagnoses typically hope for things more important to them than their own continued existence, such as reconciliation with an estranged family member or a bright future for their progeny. In counseling people professionally, and more generally, there is an obligation above all to promote conditions in which hope can flourish and to honor and support it when it emerges.

The most powerful forms of hope may not have a hoped-for object or goal at all. Both Jonathan Lear and Judith Andre have described eloquently this idea—that hope can take the form of openness to a goodness that cannot yet be named. Lear calls this "radical hope," a term he developed in recounting the story of the Crow Native American chief, Plenty Coups.[25] As the Crow culture and way of life were destroyed in the late nineteenth century, Plenty Coups retained a hope—based on a childhood vision—that something good would emerge from the devastation. Andre's term for this form of hopefulness in the face of devastation is "open hope,"[26] something rooted in a rejection of despair and in a conviction that goodness is possible that is not now known or even predictable. As Lear describes it, the hope of Plenty Coups was rooted in a spiritual tradition of sacred visions. For both Lear and Andre, hope is essentially a vulnerability to a yet-unnamed goodness that might emerge, while knowing that there is no guarantee, or even strong probability, that it will. Hope does not gain its power by relying on probabilities. Although grounded in realism, it is an openness to being surprised by goodness or what theologically is often called "grace."

7
Moral Concepts in Practice II

Voluntary and Nonvoluntary Responsibilities

To whom and for what are we responsible? One typical response is that we become responsible by explicitly making a commitment, such as making a pledge or signing a contract. For example, if I borrow money to buy a car I have a moral and legal responsibility to repay the money. Other explicit agreements, regardless of legal standing, carry full moral weight because I have committed to them. Suppose I borrow books from you and say, "I'll return these in a few weeks when I have read them." I thereby become responsible for returning the books. Even without the verbal commitment to return the books by a certain date I am responsible, since it is customarily understood that by taking your property for my own use I have incurred an obligation to return it in due course. This is what makes it a borrowing rather than the receipt of a gift. If I lose or damage it, you are owed restitution. This is the nature of accepting responsibility. Note that the responsibility is *to* someone *for* something, in this case *to* you, *for* books. In this line of thinking, it is the specifics that make it a responsibility. The obligation is voluntarily assumed. I agree to it, and the agreement can be either explicitly stated or implied by the situation.

Voluntary responsibility, based on a legal model of contracts, has an attractive feature: our responsibilities are easily knowable and are limited. If I have agreed to something, like repaying a loan or returning a book, then I am responsible for it. It follows that if I have not voluntarily assumed it, or by my actions implied it, then I have no obligation.

But life is more complicated, and things are not always as simple as this explicit contract model portrays. For example, details of assuming responsibility are often lacking and the range of obligations is vague. In marriage vows couples typically agree to love, honor, and care for each other, but without specification for just how this will occur. There is usually nothing in the vows about who will bring in what portion of the family income or how household chores will be shared. Similar vows are made at baptisms, upon joining organizations, and in many other, more routine activities. Vagueness about the exact meaning or scope of the responsibility is necessarily left to be worked out at some later time and depends on future good faith negotiations of the parties involved. If I agree to help a friend move I might say, "I'll be there by 8:00 to help load the truck," but am very unlikely to say, "I commit for a 2-hour period, with rest stops, and only for carrying boxes that weight less than 40 pounds." Unlike contracts, voluntarily assumptions of moral responsibility often carry open-ended commitments.

Most professional activities entail, simply by the nature of the work involved, assumptions of responsibility that are not named but understood as part of what the role requires. Think here of police officers, firemen, doctors, accountants, schoolteachers, public health officials, judges, holders of political office, and a host of others. All these roles assume a good faith uptake of responsibilities that normally are not named and agreed to explicitly, although they are sometimes implied in professional codes of ethics.

Some responsibilities rest on no voluntary commitment whatsoever and are a result of finding ourselves in certain life situations that we did not foresee, much less choose. In such situations our responsibilities are not involuntary, meaning done against our will, but nonvoluntary, meaning situations in which no choosing was possible. Imagine that a couple decides to have a child, but the pregnancy results in twins, or even triplets. Are the parents morally allowed to say, "We only intended and agreed to one child; we're not responsible for any others"? Here a voluntary choice (to have a child) leads to an undeniable nonvoluntary responsibility (to care for twins or triplets). Yet some situations involve no choice at all. Imagine that an elderly person needs far more help in old age, financially or physically, than anticipated. Is the adult child morally justified in saying that there is no responsibility because he didn't choose his parents, and moreover, didn't choose *this* parent, who for whatever reason needs more assistance than anyone could foresee? Adult children might say that they wish their parents had planned better or even that their parents could and should have been more prudent with their money and taken preventive measures for their health. But except for extraordinary circumstances, no adult child can say, "I didn't choose this and therefore have no responsibility to help."

Herbert Fingarette has argued that starting with voluntary responsibility is the wrong move. He believes a common, less formal kind of accepting responsibility should be the beginning of the inquiry. Instead of looking at specific acts of responsibility, we should start with the more holistic concept of a responsible person. The innovation here is that responsibility is an attribute of a person, not a feature of specific actions or choices. Being responsible is a way of life, a matter of making one's way with *know-how* through a vast array of situations and contexts, many of which are not foreseen. As Fingarette says, the responsible person "knows the ropes, although there is no rule book."[1]

Assigning responsibility is not primarily a matter of *knowing that* or enumerating just which specific actions I have selectively chosen to be accountable for. This does not mean, of course, that we will stop talking about specific acts as responsible or irresponsible, but we will ground these in something larger than personal choice. Viewing responsibility in this more complex way does leave us open to indeterminacy and thus greater vulnerability about just what the range of accountability will be. But it has the redeeming feature of being a truer description of the human situation. Much as we might sometimes desire it, none of us wants to live in a world in which responsibilities are calculated and titrated to specific contracts or promises. If a waterline in my house breaks when I am away I want my neighbor, seeing the water seeping from under my door, to at least call and tell me, not because he has promised to do so, but simply because this is what a responsible neighbor does.

The move from responsible acts to responsible persons as a beginning point explains why responsibility is a concept around which many other moral ideas turn. Not just choices, but a sense of belonging in a community and a working notion of the common good are all hinged on a robust sense of persons being responsible.

Justice and the Measure of Impartiality

Justice, we are typically told, requires the effort to see things from an unbiased view. Here bias refers to the cluster of interests and experiences that are particular to each person, and from which it is difficult to extricate ourselves. It is only natural that these particular interests and experiences that make up my perspective on the world should color my sense of right and wrong. Most understandings of justice require that we overcome or, at a minimum, rein in this narrow and provincial perspective.

One way of restraining this bias is to imagine a perspective *above* all individual interests, encompassing them, but understanding them for the partial views that they are. For some this is the view of a deity—a God's eye perspective. To work properly this divine viewpoint must include some moral teachings that emanate from this superior vantage. For example, the commandment to love one's neighbor as oneself in Christian teachings assumes that the perspective of God's love is the ultimate and final one and that it has a force and relevance beyond my particular position and the limited viewpoint I am afforded. Yet this appeal to a deity may not be convincing for several reasons. Sometimes the views of the deity and the moral teachings offered therein seem like just another limited and parochial perspective, subject to the same biases we all have. This problem becomes easier to see when we move away from teachings about love and consider the history of (supposedly) divine condemnation of, for instance, the LGBTQ communities. The closer we consider the ways this divine perspective is usually conceived and transmitted, through hierarchical religious structures and doctrines like infallibility, the more it seems that Ludwig Feuerbach was right when he said that humans have created God in their image.[2] Still, many religious people have embraced a transcendent perspective as an ideal and, in so doing, make a special point of noting that their own views fall far short.

Similarly, in the twentieth century several moral philosophers developed an imaginative device for impartiality called the "ideal observer." As Roderick Firth described and articulated it, the ideal observer is equipped with some extraordinary capacities, such as being completely knowledgeable about all the nonmoral facts of a situation, possessing an awareness of the perspectives of all parties involved, yet holding a dispassionate and disinterested stance concerning all disputing parties, as well as being perfectly logical and consistent in reasoning.[3] Firth does not imagine that anyone ever achieves this perspective. Rather it serves as a conceptual benchmark, an aspiration, and a check against subjectivity and personal bias. A judgment would then be considered right if an ideal observer would approve of it, thus providing a way of arguing for right and wrong about judgments, according to the extent that such judgments concur with or deviate from an ideal observer posture.

The chief problem with ideal observer theory is that no one ever occupies such a position, so it is hard to know when it is achieved, and perhaps even difficult to imagine. Any imaginative device that doesn't ground the moral agent in time and place may well be so idealistic as to be practically useless. It is time and place that provide for humans much of their moral orientations.

Adam Smith's device for impartiality, the "impartial spectator," instead places the individual moral actor squarely within a larger communal context—the sentiments and perspectives of others. Smith thought the point of morality was to carry each of us out of a preoccupation with our own little private world into the larger view of society:

> Though every man may, according to the proverb, be the whole world to himself, to the rest of mankind he is a most insignificant part of it. . . . When he views himself in the light in which he is conscious that others will view him, he sees that to them he is but one of the multitude in no respect better than any other in it.[4]

For Smith, internalizing this imaginative, self-effacing viewpoint of impartiality, trying to see as an impartial spectator might, is a requirement for living in society. It is also a necessity for practicing those virtues Smith considered the cardinal ones, such as justice, beneficence, prudence, and self-command. For Smith, this device of impartiality or disinterestedness was associated with a well-formed conscience.

The most prominent twentieth-century philosophical effort to achieve impartiality is the device offered by John Rawls in *A Theory of Justice*. The question of justice arises for Rawls because we all know that we have interests that will conflict with the interests of others, yet we want security and reliability in social relationships, for without these assurances social interaction would fall into a Hobbesian warlike struggle for supremacy, resulting in a life which would be, in Hobbes's words, "solitary, poor, nasty, brutish, and short."[5] Rawls's hypothetical scheme for how we ought to make such rules constitutes his distinctive contribution to the theory of justice and thus his solution to the problem of how to achieve some degree of impartiality. Imagine, he says, a starting point in which each person knows she will have interests she wants to pursue, but not specifically what these interests are. In this "original position," everyone is behind a "veil of ignorance." We do not know if we are rich or poor, with superior or inferior capacities, or healthy or sickly, and we have no sense of our social situation, our age, sex, or occupation. All we know about ourselves is that we are rational, self-interested choosers, seeking to set the rules by which society functions.[6]

Whereas Smith wants us to imagine the thoughts of others in society and Firth recommends that we imagine choosing from an all-knowing perspective, Rawls would have us choose in ignorance of our specific situation. Note that all three devices require recognition of competing interests. Yet only in Smith's impartial spectator is the imagination engaged in a concrete and situated way. His aim was not to establish a universal impartiality that either encompasses all knowledge (Firth) or strips away all self-knowledge (Rawls), but a more limited, social one—simply to imagine the way my interests are likely to be seen by others. With Firth and Rawls, I am asked to imagine a hypothetic situation for choosing; with Smith, I am asked to imagine the real perspectives of other people.

Devices for achieving impartiality are closely related to what I discuss in chapter 2 in terms of decentering. I argue that some of the most prominent of these devices in twentieth-century philosophy require either an impossible all-knowing status or a very unlikely forgetfulness of my individual situation in the world. Those that require omniscience tempt us to the same sort of moral vanity that we seek to avoid, since we are very likely to import some of our own perceptions into the definition of the universally normative one. "Wouldn't the world be better if everybody thought like I do!" we are prone to say. By contrast, those that require ignorance and forgetfulness would have us pretend that we are not historically rooted and bodily creatures. Yet because we are bodily situated beings, the particulars of our situations will be all but impossible to forget when we devise rules for a fair and impartial system.

Like all innovative devices in ethics, those seeking impartiality as a measure of justice have limits. They are very good to think with in some situations, but disastrous in others. For example, efforts at impartiality are clearly things we count on in activities such as the verdicts of judges, the calls of umpires in sporting events, the decisions of public administrators about awarding construction contracts, and professors assigning grades, among many others. Yet in other realms of moral life, impartiality seems not just useless but a vice, as many feminist moral philosophers have argued. To be sure, a parent who favored one child over another in terms of educational opportunities, other things being equal, would fail any test of impartiality, but ideal observing would be perverse if my choice is between educating my children and educating the children of strangers. Not being partial to my own children would not only go against our natural inclinations but constitute a dereliction of parental duties. That is how norms and imaginative devices for achieving impartiality sometimes become curtailed by virtues such as loyalty and the moral constraints of existing relationships. The lesson here is to choose our devices for impartiality with the same critical rigor, the same skepticism, that we bring to specific moral judgments. By so doing we will more nearly approximate justice.

Liberty and Its Limits

Liberty is etched into the American psyche in a deeper and more pervasive way than any other moral ideal. The other concepts in the trinity of the U.S. Declaration of Independence (1776)—life and the pursuit of happiness—pale by comparison and to a certain extent are anchored in liberty. Life without liberty is considered less than desirable, as in Patrick Henry's famous juxtaposition: "liberty or death."[7] And *the pursuit* of happiness in a pluralistic society is feckless and futile unless people are free.

Isaiah Berlin has provided a distinctive, twentieth-century expression of the political meanings of this key concept in his analysis of negative and positive liberty.[8] Negative liberty is essentially freedom from unwanted intrusion or control; it means freedom *from*. It is the right not to be interfered with, coerced, or controlled by the state or other powerful groups. This negative liberty is often considered a natural right and consistent with the ideas of dignity and sanctity within the private sphere of one's life. Freedom from outside interference is the logic behind the 1973 landmark ruling of the U.S Supreme Court *Roe v. Wade*, which is hinged on a right to privacy.

The generally accepted limits on this right of noninterference were articulated by John Stuart Mill. In *On Liberty* he asserts, "The only purpose for which power can be rightfully exercised over any member of a civilized community, against his will, is to prevent harm to others."[9] Known as "the harm principle," this means my right to swing my fist ends where your nose begins, my right to pollute a river is curtailed by your reliance on this water source downstream, and so on. In each case, harmful effects on others circumscribe my right to do something.

Positive liberty, as Berlin defined it, is an essential part of self-governance. It refers to the liberty to vote, choose one's leaders, and help shape the society in which one lives. Positive freedom means being able to choose those who will have moral influence and authority over me, rather than having these things foisted on me in a tyrannical way. Berlin's positive liberty is a pillar of democratic societies.

One of the great debates about the use of the harm principle in modern societies is the extent to which negative liberty should be curtailed to ensure social order. Surveillance cameras in public venues are ubiquitous in Western Europe, but less so in the United States. These are essentially invasions of privacy, or curtailments on negative liberty, justified by the goal of a safer, less crime-ridden society. The ethics of these trade-offs are routinely debated and striking the right balance in any society is a matter of considering them in the light of current realities. The U.S. populace is understandably more tolerant of surveillance after the 9/11 attacks. Nonetheless, critics of modern government penetration into the private lives of citizens in the name of security view such penetration as a potential tool of tyranny.

Autonomy, or more precisely, respect for autonomy, is the ethical synonym for the kind of liberty gains found in areas of life that in the past were controlled by experts. In these contexts, it refers to an individual's right of self-determination, even in the face of power asymmetries of knowledge and expertise. Changes in medical ethics and in human subjects research are good examples. These changes—from deference to expertise and paternalism to recognition of a right to autonomous choice—are embodied in contemporary practices of informed consent.

The legal standard for informed consent is essentially a duty of physicians to disclose information pertinent to a procedure or treatment. The ethical understanding is a more robust version of respect for autonomy. The ethical meaning of consent serves the goal not only of informing but also, as Nancy King put it, of enabling the patient to make a considered judgment based on his or her sense of what is best.[10]

In Western societies, and especially perhaps in the United States, freedom is sometimes misunderstood to entail a rejection of community. Yet the choice between individual freedom and social cohesion is a false one, famously romanticized by film stars like John Wayne and Clint Eastwood. More realistically, individual freedom is the hard-earned product of progressive, supportive communities that encourage individual flourishing.

Finally, liberty or freedom must be present as a condition for ethical engagement at all. For example, people have no choice about whether they grow hair, only whether to have it cut, curled, or dyed or to shave their heads. A penalty for growing hair—or for that matter, failing to grow it—makes no sense. Some viewers of the human situation argue that we are largely under the control of some psychological or genetic mechanism, despite the internal sense of deliberating and making choices. Seventeenth-century political philosopher Thomas Hobbes was one of these. He argued that no matter what benevolent assumptions we may have about our actions, we always choose out of self-interest. Altruism is a delusion. More recently, genetic determinists contend that genes regulate our behavior in most, possibly all, instances. Over the past two centuries, it has been argued that intelligence, social status, criminal behaviors, pyromania, and a wide range of other behaviors are determined by our genes and therefore beyond our control. I do not attempt a full refutation of determinism here. But it should be noted that in addition to being counter to human experience, deterministic philosophies are typically ideologically driven and calculated to explain why some aspect of social inequality or oppression is written into the psychological or biological code and thus "natural" and unchangeable. Blacks were typically not educated in the antebellum South, it was argued, because they did not have the intelligence to become literate. Women, it was widely argued in the nineteenth century, did not possess the reasoning capacities to vote, hold office, or manage property.

One measure of moral progress in a society is the extent to which stereotypes that deny basic liberties are unmasked as prejudicial and defeated. To the extent that liberty is denied to people, their possibilities for moral flourishing and moral accountability are also denied. Liberty, then, is not just a moral good, but the condition for doing ethics at all.

Contextualizing Rights

The moral notion of rights when translated into law and social policy has arguably been the most effective tool for advancing the welfare of the human species in the last 300 years. Yet much work remains, even within democracies, and especially in more traditional and autocratic societies.

Philosophers tend to categorize rights in a variety of ways. Some rights are thought to be natural, meaning that people implicitly possess them. Sometimes these inherent rights are designated as God-given endowments, as in the words of the American Declaration of

Independence. Whatever their origin, natural rights are "unalienable," meaning that they cannot be removed or altered. Having such rights is ordinarily what we mean when we say that people have dignity. As Immanuel Kant put it, everything either has a price or a dignity.[11] Anything with a price can be replaced, but things with dignity are beyond monetary calculation or market exchange.

Conventional rights, by contrast, refer to specific civil and social powers granted by political institutions, such as the U.S. Constitution's Bill of Rights (1791), guaranteeing, for example, the right of freedom of speech, assembly, and worship.

Like freedom, rights can also be negative or positive. Negative rights are essentially rights of noninterference and require nothing of others except respecting our freedom and privacy. Positive rights, by contrast, require action by others and place an obligation on them to deliver. For example, my right to be free from robbery and assault is a negative right, requiring nothing from others except their restraint. My right to adequate police protection for myself and my property is a positive right, placing an obligation on others to help fund and support such protection.

One useful way to read U.S. history is as a progressive moral crusade for the rights of individuals and groups whose standing as full human beings has been denied. The modern civil rights movement dates from roughly the 1950s and has challenged voting restrictions, separate public accommodations, unequal educational opportunities, unfair housing, and a range of other inequalities. Some of the heroes of these battles for human rights for African Americans are well known and widely celebrated, such as Martin Luther King Jr. and Rosa Parks.

Another example of rights language as a vehicle for social change is the United Nations Declaration of Human Rights, adopted on December 10, 1948. The first six articles are thought to be some of the most important. They address freedom from discrimination; the right to life, liberty, and personal security; freedom from slavery, torture, and degrading treatment; and the right to recognition as a person before the law. While these and the remaining 24 basic human rights do not have the status of international law, they are widely referenced and carry substantial moral weight as standards that civilized countries should honor.

The animal rights or animal liberation movement is distinctive because its origins are largely found in academic writings. The works of contemporary philosophers Peter Singer and Tom Regan are especially noteworthy. The basis of animal rights for Singer lies in the sentience of animals—their ability to suffer. He argues that the tyranny of humans over animals is like the historical tyranny of white races over blacks, in that both frustrate the interests of the oppressed.[12] Regan argues that animals possess many human capacities that we prize, such as intelligence, memory, and a subjective life. Hence, we have duties toward them, just as we do humans.[13] Accordingly, Regan calls for an end to all animal agriculture and experiments using animals and an embrace of vegetarian practices. While attention to animal rights has affected the treatment of animals in such areas as medical research, the aim of curtailing large-scale, commercial animal farming has not been realized.

Some philosophers contend the most important moral feature of rights is their preeminence among moral concepts. As Ronald Dworkin says, rights function as trumps.[14] They have a special normative force that overrides other, less important moral considerations. For example, my views may be rude, disrespectful, and factually wrong, but ordinarily I have a right to speak them. Critics of the rights-as-trumps position sometimes argue from a communitarian stance, arguing that rights have been overused as truncheons by individuals to club their opponents into submission and thereby negate larger social goods. For example, consider the assumed rights of property owners to use water upstream to the detriment of those living downstream. Feminist critics say that the predominance of rights in ethics presupposes a male perspective that undervalues care and relationships. Clearly there are many areas of life in which rights are less important than obligations, loyalties, and other social and communal values.

An emphasis on rights over other moral concepts can run contrary to the task of moral decentering described in chapter 2. At its extreme, focusing exclusively on my rights as an individual in neglect of social or community context leads to egocentrism. Rights language needs to be tempered by other moral idioms. One way to do such tempering is to correlate rights with responsibilities. It is a useful exercise to ask oneself, for every right I have, "What is the correlate responsibility I should be aware of"? The right of free speech carries a responsibility for truthfulness and avoidance of hate speech or language that incites violence. The right to walk in the wilderness carries a responsibility not to pollute streams, start fires, or leave litter. Fitting rights-and-responsibilities into these correlative pairings reminds us that some of the most important rights are not individual enfranchisements but social constructs, that is, viable only so long as they are enacted as occasions for stewardship.

Conscience: Within—Not Above—the Moral Fray

Conscience is often given a special place in moral discourse. The usual definitions see conscience as an inner voice or deep feeling that serves as a guide for right and wrong actions. As such, conscience is closely associated with a person's moral identity, so that violating one's conscience threatens moral integrity. Social and legal adjustments to accommodate conscientious objections, for example to military service, underscore the importance of respecting conscience and solidify its status as something set apart from other moral judgments.

In contemporary American society, claims of conscience arise with increasing frequency. Some pharmacists are reluctant to dispense

Plan B contraception because they think it implicates them in abortion. The consciences of some physicians steer them away from reproductive services, while other physicians are conscientiously led to provide such services. Each year a few hospital staff opt out of safety requirements, such as required vaccines for influenza, because they are conscientiously opposed to them. Parents occasionally use conscience as the moral rationale for not vaccinating their children and, sometimes, for blocking their children's access to needed therapies. And health care is not the only arena in which appeals to conscience are increasingly prominent. Think here of florists refusing to provide flowers for gay and lesbian weddings or the county clerk in Kentucky who in 2015 made a religiously informed conscientious stand against issuing marriage licenses to gay and lesbian couples.

On a personal level, most of us can clearly recall times in which conscience steered us clear of trouble when we were morally flummoxed. Yet conscience can be a guide not only into good actions, but also into evil ones. Many appeals to conscience deserve our moral respect and approbation; others represent profound moral mistakes and sometimes even corruption that merit condemnation rather than praise. In the former category, think of the nonviolent protests of Mohandas Gandhi and Martin Luther King Jr. or, more recently, NFL quarterback Colin Kaepernick kneeling during the national anthem as a protest of police violence against African Americans. In the latter category think of Robert E. Lee, Confederate military commander, who was led by conscience to violate his sworn duty to the United States to fight for succession and defend the practice of slavery.

One vivid and memorable example of the corruption of conscience occurs in *Huckleberry Finn*. Here I am relying on Jonathan Bennett's analysis of this classic Mark Twain novel.[15] As the story unfolds, Huck develops a deep attachment to Jim, a runaway slave. Together they raft down the Mississippi River toward a location where Jim will be free. As they near the end of the raft journey Huck has an attack of conscience, a conscience uncritically shaped by the slave-owning society of rural Missouri. As Bennett interprets it, the choice Huck finally makes—to help Jim escape to freedom—is one in which his affection for and friendship with Jim overcome the promptings of a racist conscience. Our own consciences, like Huck's, have their origins in childhood, in our parents and friends, in local neighborhoods, and in the schools, jobs, and religious organizations in which we find ourselves. Like Huck's, our consciences are often no better than the dominant influences of our familial, social, and religious life.

One of the interesting features of this example is that Huck is not a mature person at the time his compassion for Jim trumps his conscience. A useful exercise would be to imagine a continuation of Huck's moral development, and not end the story with Huck nursing a guilty conscience as he goes off to his next adventure.

Much of the trouble with conscience comes because of its privileged status. In moral conversations, appeals to conscience are often seen as conversation stoppers. It is as if the conscientious objector is saying, "This is how I feel, and you have no right to ask me to think further or suggest I might be wrong." Yet when conscientious objection is honored reactively it tends to value earnestness over moral insight and sincerity over careful reflection. The result is a truncated moral framework that reinforces a personal, and largely privatized, moral certitude. Because claims of conscience frequently go unexamined, they remove from play the other elements of ethical deliberation. The critical intelligence and skepticism routinely employed in other facets of ethical thinking seem to be dormant when claims of conscience are put forward. While few of us accept flaws in logic, limited empathies, a truncated imagination, or a careless use of empirical data in ethical discussions, we now tend to grant a credulous authority to conscience. About the most that is usually said is that actions of conscience should not injure others or infringe on their rights. In this way conscientious actions are not directly challenged; rather, arguments are made to circumscribe their impact. Otherwise they are to be honored, or at least tolerated. This short-circuits moral inquiry.

One reason for privileging conscience and giving it a trusting deference is because it is often closely associated with individual freedoms. Freedom of conscience is seen by many as the last stronghold against an oppressive majority or big-brother government. Following this logic, individual liberty requires a liberty of personal conscience, demanding nothing of others but tolerance and forbearance. But this libertarian mode of reasoning leaves out important substantive questions: How *should* a conscience be formed? How *should* it work? How can we *reasonably differentiate* between those promptings of conscience that should be followed and those that should not?

If a person's conscience is thought to be religiously informed, it can be understood as "the voice of God"—an unassailable authority that guards not only moral judgments but guarantees our personal moral identity and integrity. Committing acts forbidden by a divinely authorized conscience, it is thought, can destroy the whole edifice of moral self-understanding. The belief that operations of conscience are both the sharpest mirror and the final register for who one is, deep down, explains both the urgency and felt vulnerability of persons as they make appeals to conscience. Yet this fear of placing the moral self in jeopardy works to restrict the examination of what is being claimed. The idea that conscience is the final register for moral identity is no protection from its corruption. The authority it has does not come with a fail-safe device and treating conscience as an unimpeachable gift from the divine can become a recipe for moral intransigence and often for violence, as modern terrorism has tragically illustrated.

Ironically, putting conscience on a pedestal free from critical inquiry makes it more susceptible, not less, to corruption. At a bare minimum, it seems clear that tasking conscience with the maintenance of moral integrity does not insulate it from error. It does not mean that conscience can't be weak, shaped by cruel or depraved sentiments, fed by anger and hatred, impervious to empathic correction, or otherwise highly compromised by a range of vices, both moral and intellectual. My criticisms are not aimed at conscience per se, but at the presumption that conscience is a unique organizing and defining capacity for the moral self, the guardian and guarantor of integrity. A better view is that moral integrity is not a state vouchsafed by some special capacity, like a conscience, but a hard-won and fragile achievement that comes from using a range of ethical skills, such as those described in chapters 2 and 3. One thing that helps in that achievement is a commitment to acknowledge the inherent fallibility of all our moral capacities, and subsequently all the conclusions we reach, even those of conscience. This commitment means that we must share and test our moral reasoning not only within our supportive and nurturing communities but in extended conversation with those who differ.

How Death Enables Ethics

The human mortality rate is 100 percent. All lives end, but only humans have the capacity to foresee this and understand its inevitability. This recognition of finitude—that our lifespan may be long but not infinite—is fundamentally tied to human ethical capacities. To be sure, not just ethics is bound in this way to the recognition of finitude. Some of our central values—aesthetic and spiritual, as well as ethical—have little meaning in a life without limits.

Emily Dickinson spoke of this link between the defining experiences in life and our finite existence when she wrote, "That it will never come again is what makes life so sweet."[16] The poem continues in Dickinson's assertion that any consolation of an afterlife or escape from death, if it existed, would be merely a shadow of our present joy and that this thought makes her cherish the singularity of this life even more. Wallace Stevens, in his poem *Sunday Morning*, put it succinctly: "Death is the mother of beauty."[17]

One of the classic scenes of recognition of the connection between moral choices and human finitude is found in Homer's *Odyssey*. In one of the many travails of his journey home from the Trojan War, Odysseus finds himself shipwrecked on the island of the goddess Kalypso. She is beautiful, rich, and powerful and offers Odysseus a transition from his mortal state to a life of eternal bliss with his needs and appetites satisfied. Yet we find Odysseus turning his back to immortality and these endless pleasures and pining for Ithaca and his devoted wife Penelope. Kalypso's entreaties to Odysseus reveal all the hardships she foresees that he is fated to yet encounter on his journey, and she reminds him that what she is offering in beauty and sexual prowess is unequaled by any mortal woman. Odysseus answers her thus:

> Goddess and queen, do not be angry with me. I myself know that all you say is true and that circumspect Penelope can never match the impression you make for beauty and stature. She is mortal after all, and you are immortal and ageless. But even so, what I want and all my days I pine for is to go back to my house and see my day of homecoming.[18]

Why would Odysseus forgo immortality and life with a beautiful goddess and return to a dangerous voyage in hopes of reuniting with an aging spouse? The answer lies in the meaning-making capacities of a mortal life that are not available to timeless gods and goddesses.[19] Only beings who live in history, and whose personal history is limited, can find the sweetness and beauty of which Dickinson and Stevens speak. Kalypso, being immortal, lives outside time and will have an endless number of occasions for love and happiness. She cannot long for something passing, something fragile in herself, as mortals do. These beauties, and sorrows, lie beyond her. For Kalypso things come not once as they do for mortals, but eternally, so neither the fragility of beauty nor the vulnerability of goodness is available to her. Martha Nussbaum has expressed this definitively: "The peculiar beauty of *human* excellence just *is* its vulnerability."[20]

Ethics matters only if we make our choices and actions matter, in a limited world in which we have no guarantee of goodness and happiness. We do not have the power to remake our choices and lives over and over again, in endless possibility. To take a common example, a commitment to love and honor "'til death do us part" has no meaning if death never occurs. Ethics thus depends upon finitude and a recognition of this fact; that our lifespan is necessarily, and not just accidentally, limited. Because death is not simply the end result of our life but our telos—our aim or purpose—it is not just where life does lead, but where it is meant to lead. And this limited span makes things possible but not inevitable. In love, in beauty, and in ethics, the boundaries create whatever meaning is available.

The idea that limits in life help to create the moral significance of our actions does not, however, eliminate the fear of death, which remains a major impediment to our happiness. For this problem, the teachings of late Roman Stoicism are helpful. Seneca, Epictetus, and Marcus Aurelius all believed that the fear of death was the chief obstacle to freedom. Seneca, a chief advisor to the Roman emperor Nero, summarized the Stoic teachings: "He who has learned to die has unlearned slavery."[21] Michel de Montaigne, deeply influenced by the Roman Stoics, has extended passages in his *Essays* drawn from the Stoic stream. He thought the fear of death a natural part of the human make-up, but pointless and foolish.

> What stupidity to torment ourselves about passing into exemption from all torment! As our birth brought us the birth of all things, so will our death bring us the death of all things. Wherefore it is as foolish to lament that we shall not be alive a hundred years from now as it is to lament that we were not alive a hundred years ago.[22]

The good that comes from managing this fear of death is a new form of freedom and a deeper appreciation for the life one has been given. Hence, the Stoic teaching that to learn to die is to learn to live fully.

* * *

Readers will want to take up the conversation at this point, to ask about the moral concepts I have not considered. My own moral history is inescapably threaded through the discussion of each concept, just as it was in my selection of these ideas and not others. Given that we are all working out of our unique moral histories, with their own twists and turns, challenges and resolutions, no list could ever be complete. If this list has provoked readers to do their own thinking, I have achieved my aim.

8
Skills and Concepts for Ethics beyond the Lifespan

What are our responsibilities for a future we will not live to see? How should we think, ethically, about a world that will not include us? Environmentalists are now asking these questions with regularity. For example, they demand that we think about the severity of storms and droughts predicted to occur in the second half of the twenty-first century, if not sooner, and consider which of the low-lying land masses will be under water as the polar ice caps continue to melt.

Some of these events, and perhaps the most severe consequences, will occur after many of us are dead. Others of us will likely live to see some very severe effects. One of the difficulties is knowing just how quickly the changes will occur, but a recent United Nations report from a group of 91 scientists from 40 countries is very sobering.[1] The report concludes that the earth may well be in crisis as early as 2040, with accelerating wildfires, drought, and accompanying food shortages; intensified storms; and inundated coasts that will displace as many as 40 million people worldwide. The result will be drastic increases in poverty, disease, and death, overwhelming social support and health systems. A 2018 report on climate change from 13 U.S. federal agencies echoes these dire predictions. Without substantial steps to slow global warming, as much as 10 percent of the American economy will be wiped out by 2100. This would be more than twice the size of the damage from the Great Recession.[2]

Skills and Concepts in the Context of Global Warming

In considering global warming and its destructive effects, each of the skills discussed in chapters 2 and 3 should be brought into play. Let me illustrate by considering each skill briefly.

Probing skill: We have not only an individual prehistory but a collective one. The dominant moral assumptions we have imbibed see our planet as here for human advancement and pleasure. Interrogating our collective prehistory means moving beyond these assumptions to a sense of interdependence with the biosphere.

Decentering skill: Taming moral vanity and recognizing others does not mean simply including other people within our moral concerns; it can also mean other life forms which are dependent upon the health of the environment. One of the life forms to include is Earth itself.

Relinquishing skill: Giving up the comforts of moral certainty means also giving up several kinds of false assurances about environmental degradation. Among these erroneous assurances are that what we do to the environment doesn't matter and can be harmlessly absorbed; that there is no way to achieve wide cooperation for environmental improvement; that we can rely on our ingenuity for a scientific fix; and that it is too late to do anything meaningful. None of these things are certain, but acting as if they were will further paralyze us morally.

Emotional skill: What is required in terms of emotional skill is an honest recognition of our deep affective allegiance to our planet. While we cannot directly have the awe-inspiring perspective afforded the astronauts from outer space, looking at the blue orb we call "home," we can still perceive the beauty and mystery of belonging to Earth as our nurturing abode.

Cognitive skill: Fast thinking puts us in the wrong cognitive mode for environmental matters, as for most moral questions. What we can achieve in fulfilling our responsibilities to Earth is not available unless we slow down, overcome our denial, our panic, and our proclivity for quick fixes. It has taken hundreds of years of abuse to get us to this hazardous point. It will take many decades of sustained effort, over the lifespans of many generations, to remedy our situation.

Imaginative skill: Is our empathy only available to other humans, or can it stretch to other life forms, such as other animals, trees, flowers, and rivers? Even a cursory look at writers like Wordsworth, Coleridge, or Whitman suggests that our powers for empathic connections can extend to the natural world and may have no boundaries.

Assertive skill: Claiming our own moral authority in matters of environmental pollution will mean bucking the trend toward either complacency or hysterical paralysis. Here, as in other contexts, courage to own our values will be required.

Connective skill: The connection between goodness, in terms of beneficence toward the environment, and happiness is the starkest linkage imaginable, for the sort of happiness at stake is not just achieving our human potential but surviving.

Narrative skill: Responsible and concerted activity toward undoing the harm to the biosphere means rewriting the story of who we are and what we are created for—our life purpose—in relation to Earth. We humans are the only ones who can pollute the planet to this point of crisis and the only ones who can salvage it. Surely this is a moral story that supersedes all others.

What I have just sketched relating ethical skills to global warming can also be done for the interpretation of the basic concepts discussed in chapters 6 and 7. Take "the anchoring value of truth," for example. Insisting on truth-telling from our political leaders is a linchpin for collective action. But rather than describe the possible applications of each of the concepts, I raise questions for the reader about how to use these concepts. I invite readers not only to respond to these questions but to raise additional ones, and to name, describe, and apply additional concepts not discussed here.

The creation or discovery of new moral concepts, as well as skillful use of the ones listed next, can be a major resource for our survival.

The anchoring value of truth: Is candor and honesty more important when facing global warming than when dealing with other moral problems? What makes resistance to the truth so powerful a force in this context?

Forgiveness and freedom: Is forgiving ourselves and others for climate degradation more difficult than for other moral transgressions? Can forgiveness function here, as in other contexts, as an action that sets us free to reframe our responsibilities and rewrite our future?

The varieties of love: Which form of love discussed in chapter 6 is the most apt description of our affection for the planet? Do we need a new concept to describe the love for our sustaining environment? What would you call it? (See the last section of this chapter, "Getting Grounded")

The moral uses of spirituality: Do we need to consider our relation to the planet a spiritual one? Should we think of recycling as a religious act? Some Earth Day rituals already exist. Should we be incorporating them into existing religious practices?

The persistence of hope: Do we have to hope for a better future in order to envision one and work for its realization? How is "radical" hope that goes beyond a hoped-for outcome relevant to our survival?

Voluntary and nonvoluntary responsibilities: How do we enact a responsibility for the biosphere? Would you characterize this as voluntary or nonvoluntary, individual or collective? Where does it rank among other duties and obligations?

Justice and the measure of impartiality: What measures of fairness are most helpful in thinking about the biosphere? Which moral paradigms of impartiality will most forcefully energize us?

Liberty and its limits: Which freedoms must be restricted to achieve environmental aims? What positive freedom is it most important to emphasize?

Contextualizing rights: How do we conceive the rights of future generations of humans? Is it helpful for environmental understanding and action to think of rivers and trees as having rights? How should we balance rights and responsibilities in environmental matters?

Conscience: within—not above—the moral fray: The malleability of conscience suggests that care for Earth could be given a central place, becoming perhaps the most prominent urge of conscience. How might we work to enable this change?

How death enables ethics: The section in chapter 7 on death addresses individual, personal death. Can the thoughts presented there be extended to the death of homo sapiens as a species, that is, the collective "us" as well as the personal "I"? For each of us personally, the realization of our inevitable death creates ethical meaning for our life. The death of our species could bring not the creation of meaning but the end of meaning.

I argue in chapter 1 that ethics is one of the truest reflections of our humanity, a clearly discernable field of struggle for the contest between our best relational and caring selves and the more arrogant, isolated, and destructive side. If this is right, what we do about the environmental crisis at hand is the largest register imaginable of who we finally take ourselves to be.

Five Morally Debilitating Features of Our Current Thinking

As useful as these skills and concepts may be, their effectiveness is blunted by other factors when we consider environmental matters. It would be easy to blame our political leaders, especially when their denial of global warming reinforces public antiscience prejudice and serves to keep them in power. Large corporations, fixated on profit, are another easy target. But the responsibility belongs to all of us. Our current habits of thinking about ourselves and the world get in our way and short-circuit ethical reflection. In what follows I will describe five debilitating features of our current thinking and suggest an approach that could get us grounded, ethically, and free us to act.

1. Focus on the Present

When duties to people in the future are discussed, the value of those future lives is heavily discounted. Philosopher Stephen Gardiner rightly points to the intergenerational aspects of our failure to care for the environment. He argues that the "pronounced temporal dispersion of causes and effects" in climate change means that intergenerational thinking is essential to any resolution, and that "intergenerational buck-passing," with each generation locked within the confines of its own lifespan, makes the global warming tragedy unlike other tragedy-of-the-commons problems.[3] This discounting of the future was epitomized by President George W. Bush, who upon leaving office said, "I don't spend a lot of time really worrying about short-term history. I guess I don't worry about long-term history, either, since I'm not going to be around to read it."[4]

Yet for some, thinking about the future is an ever-present concern. Parents and grandparents, for example, think locally, if not globally, about their own demise and especially about the material and spiritual goods they should bequeath to their progeny. Still, their concern is typically circumscribed and limited to people they can name and to whom they have deep attachments.

Parents and grandparents are hardly alone in thinking locally and narrowly. The dominant ideas of both ethics and bioethics have done little to equip us for more global and beyond-the-lifespan thinking. The paradigms of duties and responsibilities we typically work with have severe limitations when thinking about the future, yet they could be extended in ways as suggested in the previous discussion.

2. Political Ineptness

The attempts to date to respond to our environmental predicament have not been socially or politically compelling, whether those responses have been international environmental policy, innovation in energy technologies, or even concern for our children and grandchildren. As Bruce Jennings says, the ways of talking that would allow us to express our current predicament and show a way of responding effectively are not yet a prominent part of the political landscape.[5] One difficulty is that the carbon tax approach is widely seen as an additional tax and thus punitive. David Leonhardt argues that a better approach may be the Green New Deal, which gives people a vision of what's at stake, tying environmental action with greater equality and opportunity and thus is more progressive in orientation.[6] Yet for the present, we in the United States are headed in precisely the wrong direction. President Trump has repeatedly mocked the science behind climate change and revived one of the chief carbon offenders, the coal industry. Moreover, he has announced his intention to withdraw from the Paris accord on climate change and is opposed to any form of reducing our carbon footprint. These irresponsible policies will only hasten and magnify the damage.

Dale Jamieson, an environmental scientist and philosopher, says that the weakness in our institutions to mount an effective response to our crisis reflects an evolutionary deficit. We are not equipped as a species "to address or even to recognize this kind of problem."[7] Other writers think the problem simply has yet to be engaged. Donald Brown, an environmental lawyer, observes that those against environmental regulations have succeeded in a strategy of denial. They frame the issues in ways that evade moral responsibility by focusing on the fringes of scientific opinion that are skeptical of the facts and by playing on public ignorance of science and the tendency to deny bad news.[8]

3. Humans as the Crown of Creation

An additional problem is that much of contemporary ethics is suffused with a conviction, however tacit, that humans are the moral center of the universe. Sometimes this belief shows up in the myopic assumption that humans are the only beings who live within and are defined by a web of values. At a minimum, it is the hubris that whatever values might reside in other life forms, human values will always count for more. It is only within the last few decades that animal rights have had a robust presence in Western ethics, and the sense of beneficent obligations to Earth are even more recent.

Biologist Mary Beth Saffo has put this human egocentrism elegantly, drawing from Ann Druyan: "We see our world as the endpoint of evolution," not only the center of the universe, but as "the only love object of its creator."[9] If Saffo is right, then what is required is no simple extension or adjustment of responsibility, but a turn in ethics comparable to the Copernican revolution in cosmology.

The Copernican Revolution was the paradigm shift from the Ptolemaic view of the universe, which described the cosmos with Earth stationary and at the center, to the heliocentric model with the sun at the center of our solar system. It began with the publication of Copernicus's *De revolutionibus orbium coelestium* in 1543 and reached consummation with the work of Isaac Newton over a century later. If we apply this paradigm shift to the phases of human moral development, we could say that the beginning of ethics has to do with what I describe in chapter 2 as a decentering skill—that the world does not revolve around me, but also includes other people, who have an equal or greater claim to my concern. This chastening of the ego to include others is likely grounded in the growth of several human capacities, such as abstract reasoning, imagination, and especially our capacity for empathy and the ability to imaginatively place ourselves in the shoes of others. Placing Earth rather than ourselves in the moral center is the next revolution required for our survival.

4. Consumerism

The idea that human values and needs supersede all else is tied to the influx of consumer motifs into contemporary ethics. If humans are the only species that really counts, then Earth and its natural resources, not to mention all other forms of life, can be bent to human needs and desires. One of the ways this notion shows up is in the current subservience of all other moral principles—including responsibility—to the principle of autonomy, conceived in a consumerist frame. The right to choose in the market without social or communal constraints seems to be the one value on which most Americans agree. Yet the consumerist notion of autonomy refers not to freedom from coercive social and governmental forces, as John Stuart Mill would have it,[10] but to a freedom to possess anything one can afford to buy. In the consumerist view of the world, essential values are displayed by possessions and purchasing power.[11] Instead of voting or participating in civic life, shopping and consuming is the activity that best defines us.

Religious studies scholar Jay McDaniel argues that consumerist attitudes and values "now function as an unofficial, corporate-sponsored world religion. Its evangelism occurs through advertisements, and its church is the mall."[12] McDaniel's central idea is that thinking of consumerism as a religion makes clear how a consumerist lifestyle knows no natural bounds. More is always better, and overconsumption becomes the norm. This explains why, for example, in the United States we use up such a disproportionate amount of the world's resources—40 percent of the world's fresh water and 75 percent of its energy.[13] McDaniel echoes Alan Durning's concluding question from his book *How Much Is*

Enough?: "Having fully met our material needs . . . can [we] now craft a new way of life at once simpler and more satisfying[?]"[14]

5. Mechanistic Views of Nature, Including the Human Body

The seventeenth-century French philosopher René Descartes was a champion of the mechanistic view of nature. For Descartes, the mind is a reality wholly separate from the physical body. Bodily sensation and sensory perception are distrusted—at best they are morally inert; at worst they are illusory and misleading. The only certainty comes from what we can clearly and distinctly think. Nature, including the emotions, senses, and other functions of our physical bodies, is simply not a sound source of knowledge or understanding.

Our moral habits in the twenty-first-century West are deeply Cartesian. The current environmental predicament is the nearly inevitable consequence of Cartesian tendencies. The impact these tendencies have had on ethics is nothing short of debilitating. A Cartesian approach to ethics neglects the moral senses that are available only with and through the body. Alienated from its bodily roots, a Cartesian stance discounts those tacit and subtle intimations that give us a sense of place in our world. It also diminishes respect for all forms of life.

The Cartesian approach has been, to be sure, roundly critiqued. Thomas Nagel refers to this rootless moral perspective as an "excess objectivity," since it encourages us to count as relevant only those moral understandings that can be detached from our situation and from the circumstances and the history of our place in the world. He disparagingly calls this "the view from nowhere."[15] Feminist thinkers of the past few decades have also been articulate on this point. Seyla Benhabib, for example, distinguishes between "the generalized and the concrete other," arguing that the universal standpoint is illogical and feckless.[16] The Cartesian stance has indeed historically discredited the moral experiences of women, but it has also discredited a wide range of human moral experiences more generally. It has led to an incoherent morality. It denies the very conditions that make abstract thinking possible: having a safe place *from which* to think, not to mention the physiochemical circuitry *with which* to think. The future we face is one Descartes and his like-minded disciples could not have imagined.

***

In summary, our everyday working notions of ourselves and our moral duties tend to be focused on the present, without a motivating policy language to curtail global warming, hampered by the assumption that we are the crown of creation, thereby dominated by consumerist understandings of our relation to the world and, finally, prey to mechanistic views of nature. In this ethical, social, and political environment it is not surprising that responsibility for the biosphere and all those who live within it—including ourselves—gets little traction.

Getting Grounded

We desperately need a pivot into a culture in which humans listen to the innate animal sense of belonging to the earth—physically, psychically, and morally. An ethics that speaks to the current human predicament must be grounded through bodily presence and attunement with—not above—a world that antedates us, will continue without us, and to which our very existence is intimately linked. Here the work of twentieth-century French philosopher Maurice Merleau-Ponty is particularly helpful. *Phenomenology of Perception*, his major work, is a sustained refutation of Cartesian models of perception, language, and psychology, later extended into art and political discourse. His work showed that "the perceiving mind is an incarnated mind."[17] He sought to establish the roots of the mind in a body, and the body as a living organism rooted in the world. The question his work raises for ethics is whether this connectedness, this irrevocable grounding of all human activity in bodily sentience, is to be cherished and trusted or distrusted and perhaps even denied. The most basic ethical question is thus what humans make of this bodily groundedness—and whether it evokes love and loyalty or aversion and denial.

The Pauline version of Christianity teaches a suspicion of the body and distrust about its basic needs and desires. For example, in Paul's teachings the term "flesh" refers to those desires and inclinations that alienate people from God. "Flesh" in Paul's theology is opposed by "spirit," thus institutionalizing disdain for the body and its needs and affections as a fundamental moral norm.[18] While there are other Christian interpretations of the body, the Pauline version is dominant. Plato taught a similar disregard that has also been influential in Western views of the person. In the Platonic version, the soul is prized while the body is considered of little value. The Platonic dualism of an imperishable soul yoked to a perishable, and often burdensome, body finds its modern home in Descartes's model of humanity as previously discussed.[19]

Our earthly grounding can and ought to be a loving embrace. This is the most important missing ingredient for environmental ethics. We can learn to care for the earth if we see ourselves as inextricably knotted with it in a loving intertwinement. Acknowledging this intertwining can reawaken and nurture the deep, atavistic affection that existed prior to abstract thinking. This is a love that precedes verbal expression, the love we have for our habitat as animals, that is, that we had before we turned our analytic and consumptive gaze upon the world. Stephen J. Gould, the late Harvard paleontologist and historian of science, also identified love as the central motive to save the planet. "We cannot win this battle to save species and environments without forging an emotional bond between ourselves and nature as well—for we will not fight to save what we do not love."[20] I differ from Gould only in the conviction that this emotional bond need not be forged, but simply rediscovered and acted upon.

Clues to this reawakening can be found in the writings of two important twentieth-century religious thinkers, one Jewish, the other Christian. Abraham Heschel's approach to the proper human demeanor to life and the world emphasizes awe and wonder over faith and obedience to laws: "Mankind will not perish for want of information, but only from want of appreciation."[21] In a complementary vein, H. Richard Niebuhr pinpoints the most basic ethical move of humans as trust or distrust of the fundamental powers by which we are constituted and through which the world exists.[22] These fundamental powers can be seen theologically, as Niebuhr believed, in a benevolent God, or in more evolutionary terms as the happy combination of chance and necessity that gives humans life. Or both. This trust is deeply connected to the sense of awe and wonder Heschel describes and to an affection for the world, and one's self in it, that wells up from acknowledging our earthly rootedness. Whatever reorientation of responsibility will be most relevant to our current time must be grounded in just this sort of love.[23] Oliver Sacks expresses it well in his posthumously published memoir *Gratitude*: "I have been a sentient being, a thinking animal, on this beautiful planet, and that has been an enormous privilege and adventure."[24]

If we can recapture the sense of ourselves as *privileged thinking animals* on this *beautiful planet*, there may still be time for us.

I have argued here for a renewed and more relevant understanding of our obligations, grounded in a deep love for the earth as our only habitat. This understanding can also be expressed in traditional imperative form. Ernest Callenbach has provided just that in "Earth's 10 Commandments." His formulation echoes the stress on love as the foundational dynamic. His first commandment reads, "Thou shall love and honor the Earth for it blesses thy life and governs thy survival."[25]

This sort of love and honor for Earth will be aided by the realization not just that this planet is a place on which life developed, but that life as we humans now know it is an organic extension of millions of years of Earth's life. Astrobiologist David Grinspoon said, discussing the Gaia principle developed by Lynn Margulis and James Lovelock, we should think of life not as something that happened *on* Earth, but something that has happened *to* Earth.[26] In humans, Earth becomes conscious of herself. Earth not just as a place we are enabled to have bodies but that is part of our embodiment. Both metaphorically and literally, Earth breathed its life into us. Getting grounded ethically about our relationship to Earth means that we grasp the elemental fact that we don't simply stand on Earth, we are mysteriously rooted in it. In chapter 5 I argue that one of the fundamental pitfalls in ethics is treating mysteries as problems. I would here argue that we have to recognize the mystery of awe and reverence for Earth to understand and respond to the problems we have created.

In sum, our contemporary thinking is deeply flawed, but we cannot think our way into a new relationship with the world. Rather we must open ourselves to what is already there, through how we see and hear, what we feel, what we know in our bodies, before thinking with categories and concepts. Our fundamental relationship with Earth needs to be felt before it can be thought, sensed before it can be conceptualized, loved before it becomes as real as it needs to be for us to act to save it. Our deepest sense of belonging is one of being birthed for life on an amazing and wonderful living planet. It is out of this primal sense that right thinking and right action can grow.

9
Cracking the Case, and Cases to Consider

Cracking the Case

Before reading further, write about a situation in which you personally encountered a moral question. Provide as much detail as you think necessary for a reader to get the sense of the problem and your thinking about it. We will return to this later.

* * *

Many books on ethics include cases to ponder. Sometimes these are classic cases in a field, such as the Terry Schiavo case in medical ethics[1] or the Enron case in business ethics.[2] Other texts offer hypothetical situations, some of them well known, such as the trolley problem that has fascinated experimental psychologists and moral philosophers.[3] These classic and hypothetical cases are interesting but of limited practical value, and they can lead in unproductive directions. Classic cases carry a lot of baggage in terms of commentaries and well-rehearsed resolutions. Often, we are pre-empted from doing our own thinking by knowing the way the case was resolved or what others think about it.

Hypothetical cases frequently depict choices we have not faced and likely will never face. The trolley problem is a good example. It offers dichotomous options: allowing a runaway trolley to stay on track and kill five people or diverting it to an alternative track where it kills only one. Aficionados of the trolley problem claim that it validates and repudiates some major ethical theories—that it validates utilitarianism and repudiates rule-based duties—since most people think they would choose to switch tracks to kill only one person instead of five. Yet no theory can ever be validated by a hypothetical. Theories are devised for helping people in our common world with ordinary problems, or at least problems they could conceivably face. They are not strategies for dealing with far-fetched scenarios. But it isn't just hypotheticals like the trolley problem that suffer from improbability. Classic cases as well often deal with extraordinary situations, and these exceptional circumstances are less than optimum for probing the moral sensibility of most of us. The best and most instructive cases are those reported by people reflecting on their own experiences, issues they or their friends have encountered that puzzle and perplex them. Listening to others report on their ethical issues heightens their relevance when the problems are like those we have encountered ourselves or can well imagine we might encounter. That is why I asked you to begin this section by writing about a morally perplexing situation from your own experience.

In dealing with any ethics case, the first task is to interrogate the presentation itself, that is, the terms in which the situation is offered as a moral issue. The following two situations offer opportunities to reflect on how cases inevitably carry framing issues and assumptions. The cases are simple ones, but reflecting on the assumptions behind them can prepare us for dealing with more complex ones and for approaching both classic and hypothetical cases with greater awareness of just how they are being presented. Even more than "solving" the case, this kind of probing provides occasions for moral insight.

Case 1: A patient is brought to the emergency department (ED) in impending shock. The diagnosis is laceration of the liver with internal bleeding. From listening to the assessment of the ED physicians, you surmise that his chances of survival are quite slim. The patient's personal physician is called but is a long way from the

ED, and this patient seems to have identified you, a volunteer assisting in the ED, as someone to confide in. The patient is still conscious and alert as you are helping to wheel him into the operating room. Just as the cart is about to roll through the swinging doors, the patient asks you, "Doc, am I going to make it?" What should you say?

Case 2: Frank Atkinson, age 45, suffered a high vertebral fracture while horseback riding on his ranch. The accident left him paralyzed from the neck down. Mr. Atkinson was an eager participant in rehabilitation, and he had a close family with enough financial resources to provide a wide range of rehabilitative and support services. During a three-year period following the accident, Mr. Atkinson considered his life "challenging, but worthwhile." Then a series of repeated infections and hospitalizations marked the beginning of a change in his quality of life. Following the most recent hospitalization, Mr. Atkinson voiced a growing conviction that "the flame isn't worth the candle anymore," and he requested readmission to the hospital to have his respirator removed, be given sedation, and allowed to die. Should Mr. Atkinson be readmitted and helped to die?

Several features of these cases stand out immediately. For example, in Case 1, the reader is provided an assigned role and is specifically addressed for a response. The information is scant and largely impressionistic. The facts are little more than what an untrained person can "surmise." Additionally, as a volunteer, the responder has, at best, the role of an assistant, wheeling patients into the operating room, and perhaps most important, you as the respondent are foisted into a role you did not seek and are not qualified to fulfill, by a severely wounded and anxious patient you do not know.

This case is a vehicle for unearthing assumptions of all sorts, for example, assumptions about what role can legitimately be assumed by a volunteer in this context. Some students to whom I have posed this case begin their responses with a clarification that corrects the patient's mistake, saying, "I'm not a doctor." Others think a truthful response to the patient's question, wrapped in some reassurance, is called for, such as, "You are seriously injured, but our surgeons are great." Others prefer, "You have a chance," or to buff up what is thought to be a placebo response, "You have a good chance," or even, "You're going to make it." This leads to the issue of truth-telling—probing the question of to whom and on what occasions we are tempted to lie, and when, if at all, it is justified. (The moral significance of truth is considered in chapter 6.)

Case 2 is also presented by an unidentified narrator. Yet unlike Case 1, here the reader is provided a sketch of the patient, and a sympathetic one, as we learn that Mr. Atkinson has sought to end his life in a humane fashion only after a long struggle and with at least some deliberation about the quality of life he can now tolerate. The reader, without any identifying role assignment, is asked what should be done. So, we don't know if the respondent is a neutral observer or a serious stakeholder in the case, for example, a physician or nurse who could be involved in carrying out Mr. Atkinson's wishes or, say, a hospital board member or a relative of Mr. Atkinson, to name just a few possibilities. And knowing this would, of course, make a difference. One might well imagine that any of these individuals would have written this case differently and thereby embarked on a quite different fact-finding, reflective, and deliberative moral process. For example, a physician or nurse might well ask whether this request is in keeping with their professional role as specified in oaths or codes of ethics. A hospital board member would likely be concerned with liability and/or the hospital's reputation. Although it looks as if Case 2 has a more "objective" construction, as it is not addressed as a problem to anyone in particular; it is just this idea of objectivity in case construction that needs examining. "Cracking the case" means precisely this effort to interrogate not just the case but its formulation and presentation, recognizing that this case—like all cases—could well have been portrayed in a wide variety of ways. Regarding both Cases 1 and 2, we need to ask, What assumptions inform the terms in which the moral problem is couched? What questions are begged? Whose perspective is privileged, and whose is ignored?

Notice that even the term "case" suggests a somewhat arbitrary limit on what experiences will count as relevant—an encasement, suggesting perhaps a final or definitive formulation. It is useful here to remember that in its common uses outside of ethics a case is a container for convenience, for toting around things in manageable units that we would otherwise find difficult to transport, such as a violin case. Another use of "case" refers to the framing for a window: the casing, implying a viewing that enables but is also selective and restricted. Of course, some restrictions and limitations are inevitable. This is not an argument for bathing in an endless stream of moral consciousness or unending fact-gathering, which would be debilitating, but it is an argument for a recognition of the limitations of any framing of events.

Consider, for example, the varieties of ways ethics cases can and are used in teaching exercises and popular media and the extent to which they become selective instruments in the process:

- *To illustrate the features of a particular kind of moral problem.* Sometimes cases are constructed to represent important or frequently occurring problems. For example, Case 1 is representative of the temptations to deviate from truth-telling, and Case 2 is illustrative of the difficulty in finding a supportive place for a timely death.
- *To present a classic conundrum for readers to ponder.* In some cases, the "right" answer is still a matter of contention. These cases are typically truncated or manipulated during their construction to drive the reader to a point of choice, such as Case 1. This manipulation can be combined with an effort to demonstrate that no ethical judgment should be attempted in

rushed or emergency situations. Here the lesson might be to use your best instincts; the important point is to learn from this experience and devise a morally sound strategy for similar situations in the future.
- *To present a particularly good or a particularly bad example of moral reasoning.* For example, if we alter Case 2 so that the physicians refuse to admit Mr. Atkinson and assist in his death, we might intend the case to illustrate impoverished medical-legal reasoning that does not sufficiently consider the patient's plight at end of life.
- *To probe the depth and complexity of moral experience itself.* Cases can be constructed to remind us that our view is frequently opaque. For example, in Case 2, Mr. Atkinson is going through experiences that few of us will have, and this becomes a lesson in the importance of an expansive empathy to realize the magnitude of his suffering.
- *To present allegories for principles.* Cases can be and often are constructed to illustrate the importance or pre-eminence of some principle or another, to help that principle stand out in our moral repertoire. For example, with a few more sympathetic details, Case 2 can be seen as an allegory for patient autonomy, so that the reader is invited to praise any actions that help Mr. Atkinson and condemn any actions that inhibit him as paternalistic.

In each of these instances, persons and events are framed for our use. This practice is not necessarily wrong since some framing is inevitable, but every framing can also be limiting and distorting. The remedy is not to stop constructing cases, but to be aware of when, how, and why we are constructing them as we do, and the liabilities of doing so. Cases give us ways to get around the difficult terrain of ethical work, and they present the work of ethics in manageable units, and for this they are enormously useful. Without cases, we would be carrying around our ethical violins in awkward and cumbersome ways. But notice that the case is a mere container for the instrument, and it is the instrument that must be played. The exciting stuff doesn't happen when the instrument is in the case, but only after we take it out. Imagine a violin case that could be only partially opened, and only those compositions that were possible within these limitations could be performed.

To better illustrate the limits of knowledge in framing a presentation, let me move to another metaphor. The casing of moral experience is like map-making—likely to both orient and to distort, depending on how the map is used. Think, for example, of a Mercator projection map, very likely the sort hanging on the classroom wall throughout your elementary education. It represents the spherical globe as a flat surface with longitudinal and latitudinal lines all meeting at right angles. This perspective greatly exaggerates land masses at the polar regions, making them appear much larger than they are. It is a very unhelpful map if your purpose is to compare the relative size of land masses. But it is a very clever one if your aim is to be able to chart a nautical course in a straight line, which was the great advantage that Gerardus Mercator, the Flemish cartographer, had in mind for explorers in the sixteenth century.

Imagine now the task of devising a useful map of the city in which you live. Such a map could be drawn by driving the streets from a variety of directions, in which case one would be likely to include in the map the location of gas stations, the size and condition of roads, and so on. But a pedestrian map would be quite different, as would a map for antique collectors, tennis players, or educators, who might well want to know the location of the good coffee shops and bookstores.

The theme here is Aristotelian: cases are constructed by moral agents for specific purposes. A "good" case in this limited sense is one that serves its purpose well. Judgments about the quality of cases presuppose identifying the ends and purposes sought in case construction, as well as discernments about skillful use of the cases themselves. But granting the usefulness of cases does not mean we don't need to critically examine their frames. So while granting the variety of ends and purposes to which cases can be put, some generic features of good framings can be provided. For example, cases that strive for accuracy about the facts and attribute genuine moral agency—the ability to judge right from wrong—to the actors described in the cases will serve us better than those that do not. Cases that merely sketch or caricature motivations and intentions are inferior to those that provide a more robust portrait of these factors. Case constructions that seek to locate the moral actions in social and familial contexts and rely less on stereotypes are better than those that fail to do so. One of the most fatal mistakes in ethics is failing to interrogate the case and naively taking the initial framing of the ethical problems and people it presents as definitive or final. Tod Chambers has written eloquently about the fictive dimensions of all ethics case presentations, and his summation of his work is an apt one for the case "cracking" I emphasize here. "When ethicists write cases, they are rhetorically imposing a world upon us, a world that excludes as well as includes those particularities that allow us to make the best possible moral decisions."[4] Chambers urges attention to the rhetoric of cases, more careful reading, and a recognition that there are always other ways of seeing and writing.

* * *

Go back now to the case you wrote before reading this section. Did you write in the first person or the third person? Is your voice active or passive? Are you the chief protagonist? Perhaps the victim? Are the persons in the problematic situation richly described or only thinly as stick figures or placeholders? Are the motives and intentions of the characters involved attributed fairly? Can you imagine that the case could be rewritten into several different versions, from different points of view? Are the options for resolution presented with an even hand? Are they truly the only options?

Can you rewrite your morally problematic situation in light of what you have learned in this section? Asking these questions will not necessarily enable us to reach a better conclusion, but it will enable us to ask better questions and frame these and future cases in more realistic and productive ways.

Cases to Consider
(or to Rewrite as Cracked Cases)

The following cases are drawn from a very wide range of experiences and situations. Some are concerned with students of various ages, some with professionals, and some with matters of policy addressed to the public. But regardless of to whom they may immediately apply, each case has potential for sharpening our moral awareness and for practicing dexterous use of the skills and concepts described in this book. For each case, in addition to the questions listed, consider the following:

- Which relational skills, as described in chapters 2 and 3, would have prevented this problem, and which relational skills are most needed to resolve it?
- Which concepts, as described in chapters 6 and 7, are most relevant to productively framing this situation and probing it ethically?

1. Adderall for Nonprescription Uses

Adderall is a central nervous system stimulant used to treat attention-deficit/hyperactivity disorder (ADHD). At regular therapeutic doses addiction is unlikely. However, at high recreational doses, drug dependence and addiction are far more likely. Because of its addictive potential, Adderall is a Schedule II controlled substance in the United States, available only by prescription from a physician.

Students at Distinguished University ask their classmates and roommates with legitimate, prescribed ADHD possession of Adderall to give them a few pills to help with difficult periods in the semester, especially during final exam time. The students requesting the Adderall claim that it keeps them more fully alert during exams and able to perform at a higher level under stress. They justify such usage as "harmless," and they contend that "everybody does it."

- Is nonprescription use of Adderall morally OK? Are the students right to claim that such use is "harmless"? Does it matter how many other students may also be doing it?
- How would such nonprescription provision of Adderall affect the friendship of the students who request it and those who provide it?
- Should Distinguished University prohibit and punish nonprescription use of Adderall among its students (e.g., by writing a prohibition into the university's honor code)?

2. Programming a Self-Driving Car

Self-driving cars, it is said, will make the roadways safer, reducing accidents and saving lives. Since computers do not become drowsy, distracted, or drunk, they should be embraced as a great advance in highway travel. Yet, in some situations, they raise moral issues about how they should be programmed. For example, in congested traffic situations in which several vehicles and pedestrians are involved, avoiding a crash may be impossible and injuries or even fatalities likely. Imagine a situation in a crowded urban intersection in which the computer controlling the steering and breaking systems must be programmed to either protect the driver of the car or groups of pedestrians. In such cases, the human judgment is eliminated from the immediate situation of an impending accident, but the strategic judgment—a moral one—is programmed into the default mechanisms of the vehicle.

- What would be the benefits and liabilities of a simple utilitarian calculus—saving the most lives or doing the least amount of harm—as the best way to program a self-driving car?
- Imagine a car that typically carries not only one passenger but a family with children. Car owners might argue that they owe first loyalty to their families and to jeopardize their families in deference to the safety of strangers on the highway is wrong—an abandonment of parental duties. How plausible is this moral reasoning?
- What if the self-driving vehicle is not a car but a city bus or a school bus? How does this change the situation ethically?

3. Buying and Selling Organs

Currently, it is illegal to buy and sell human organs in the United States. While donation of organs is encouraged, a market for organs has been banned since 1984. Most industrial democracies have similar policies. Lester Dunkirk, an impoverished but healthy 23-year-old, wants to sell one of his kidneys to help his parents and to assist him in paying for training in auto mechanics. Most people can sustain their health adequately with only one functioning kidney, and there is every reason to think that Lester is typical in this respect.

Lester argues that it's his kidney, and he should be able to do what he wants with it. He also argues that someone needing a kidney would be helped through the sale. Those opposed to a market for organs typically argue that people like Lester will be exploited and that their poverty puts them at high risk for making poor choices about their health. Others claim that a market for organs is an assault on human dignity.

- Many things are for sale in our society, including some body parts such as hair, eggs, and sperm. Is the sale of a kidney different? If so, what makes it different?
- Would a carefully regulated market for solid organs help to overcome the objections? For example, it has been suggested that a market in which one could sell but not buy would eliminate a price war that favors the rich and still increase the supply of organs for those in need. For example, a government agency could set a price for organs and disallow bidding and also control the distribution as it currently does under the United Network for Organ Sharing. This way Lester could sell his organ without a bidding war, and the decision about who would receive it would be made through a fair process of allocation. Would such a regulated market solution resolve the problems?

4. Businesses That Provide Services Selectively

Restaurants near beaches and ballparks sometimes refuse service to customers without shirts or shoes. Some upscale establishments refuse service to male diners without a jacket. But how far should such selection of customers go? Should florists or bakers be able to say categorically that they will not provide services to people whose lifestyles or personal choices they disapprove of? Some merchants have claimed that they should be free to decline to provide their goods and services to gay or interracial weddings. While there may be prudent public health rationales for refusing service to a sweaty shoeless or shirtless customer in a restaurant, weddings pose no such public health hazard. Peter Morrison is a baker in Detroit famous for his wedding cakes. For originality of design and culinary quality, he has no peer. But he refuses to bake for customers he knows or suspects to be atheists, going so far as to refuse his services to any who marry in civil ceremonies, rather than religious ones. Peter attributes the high divorce rate to what he terms "an increasingly Godless culture," and while he admits he is losing some business because of these restrictions, he insists, "I bake the cakes and can sell them to whom I want."

- Is Peter Morrison's selective sales policy morally OK?
- How would your moral assessment of Morrison's policy change if he were refusing services to persons of Italian descent, or those who were significantly overweight, or those couples whose age difference was more than 15 years?
- What about a gourmet restaurant that refuses to serve steak well done, irrespective of its customers' preferences?
- Imagine that Peter Morrison is not a baker but a nurse, a physician, or a pharmacist. Would a conscientious objection about serving a certain group of people look different morally if the service provider is a health professional?

5. The Magnifying Effects of Social Media

Susan, a 17-year-old female high school student, has been dating her classmate Shane, also 17, for several months when he decides he no longer wants to date her. She is crushed and goes to her Facebook account to describe to her many Facebook "friends" what has happened. In her disappointment and sorrow she embellishes the relationship, claiming it was more intimate than it was and falsely stating that she was forced into unwanted sexual familiarity by Shane. Almost immediately Shane begins to receive emails and calls expressing disgust at his supposed behavior, some of them threatening.

- What should you do if you were a friend of Susan, or of Shane, or both?

- How should the parents of Susan and Shane respond and what strategies might they use?
- What moral stake, if any, do Facebook and other social media platforms have in how their platforms are used?

6. Choosing the Sex of One's Children

John and Mary Clark have two boys, John Clark Jr. (Johnny) and Frank. They desperately want a girl to "balance their family." With this in mind, Mary Clark chooses an obstetrical service that she knows is willing to do a wide range of prenatal tests, many of them for early diagnoses of diseases, but also including early identification of the sex of a fetus. After much discussion, the clinicians agree to terminate an otherwise healthy fetus if it turns out to be another boy.

- Setting aside any legal concerns, should the Clarks be able to abort a fetus based on its sex? If you think not, what would count as a weighty enough reason to justify an abortion? If you believe that this is well within the range of choices to which Mary Clark is entitled, are there any limits on what choices she might ethically make about termination?
- Imagine that the Clarks' goal is not to have a girl but to produce a sibling that would be a genetic match for Johnny, who suffers from a rare blood disorder that could be treated by transplant of umbilical cord blood from a sibling with a very close genetic resemblance to him. In this variation, the Clarks would contribute sperm and ova for in vitro fertilization (IVF), in which an extracted egg is fertilized by sperm in a laboratory, outside any human body. The obstetrics practice would then screen the embryos for genetic resemblance to Johnny, implanting in Mary Clark only those embryos that bear sufficient genetic resemblance to Johnny. Is this idea of seeking to create a "savior

sibling" less ethically troubling, or even more troubling, than aborting a fetus on the basis of its sex?

7. Vaccine Refusal: Personal Health and Public Health

Human papillomavirus (HPV) is a very common sexually transmitted disease, and about a quarter of females in the 14 to 24 age range carry an HPV infection. In the 20 to 24 age range, the infection rate exceeds 40 percent. In most of these cases the infection clears within a few years, but the remainder are at high risk for cancer of the cervix, with roughly 11,000 new cases annually in the United States. For the past several years an effective vaccine for HPV has been available, and the Centers for Disease Control and Prevention (CDC) and other medical groups have urged patients to get this vaccine.

Dawn and Jason Woodbine are the parents of a 13-year-old daughter, Molly. After a conversation with their pediatrician Dawn and Jason declined the HPV vaccine for Molly. It is not needed, they insist, since Molly is not sexually active and has been taught to abstain from sexual activity before marriage.

- Are the Woodbines making a responsible choice for their daughter?
- Do you think the Woodbines can be confident about their belief that Molly is not now sexually active and will remain so until marriage?
- What should Molly's pediatrician do if Molly tells the pediatrician in confidence that she has no personal investment in abstaining from sexual activity prior to marriage and would like to receive the HPV vaccine? What if Molly were 16 years old, told her pediatrician in confidence that she already was sexually active, and wanted to receive the HPV vaccine?

- HPV can infect males as well as females. The disease consequences are usually less severe, but cancer of the penis or the esophagus is a possibility, and the probability of these increases with the number of sexual partners. In addition, male-to-female transmission is a more likely vector of infection than female-to-male. Would you support mandatory HPV vaccinations for both males and females?
- Vaccine refusal by parents for their children has increased over the past decade and now includes routine childhood vaccines for measles, pertussis, diphtheria, and tetanus. Often this refusal is based in an erroneous belief that such vaccines can cause autism. Do parents have a right to refuse vaccines based on false beliefs when such refusals can compromise the health of other children, as well as their own?

8. Cows and Global Warming

In 2016, the average American consumed 56 pounds of beef. Worldwide, the consumption of beef was just short of 26 billion pounds. But our consumption of steaks, roasts, and burgers comes at a high cost for the environment. An average cow releases between 70 and 120 kilograms of methane a year. It is estimated that methane has a negative effect on the biosphere 23 times greater than the effect of automobile exhaust and is responsible for about 18 percent of all greenhouse gases. The world's total cow and bull population exceeds 1.5 billion, or roughly one bovine for every five people on earth. Milk production is also a factor in the bovine population problem. In 2017 Americans drank 98 metric tons of milk, with worldwide consumption more than five times that amount.

- Should Americans practice and promote little or no beef and milk consumption? In addition to the methane issue, beef is a form of protein that is very costly to produce. A healthy diet

without beef and dairy is achievable but requires considerable effort. In light of global warming and the degradation of the biosphere, should abstinence from beef and dairy consumption be considered a moral obligation? Even a diet that is beef-free, but not dairy-free would help. Should this less stringent diet be a moral goal?
- Should government programs be instituted that aim to make beef-free and/or dairy-free diets the new social norm? Surtaxes on these products at the point of purchase would be one option, while barriers to cheap meat and dairy production would be another. Do either of the alternatives make sense morally?

9. Age as a Screen for Expensive Therapies

With progress in medicine over the past four decades, it has become increasingly safe to transplant vital organs (hearts, lungs, kidneys, and livers) from deceased donors to living recipients; concurrently, recipients can now expect (on average) more and more years of extended life thanks to their donated organs. But there are far fewer donated vital organs available than there are potential recipients who could benefit from a donated organ, and the transplant process is very expensive. Some bioethicists have argued that transplanted vital organs should not be made available to people of advanced age, such as those who reach 75 or 80.[5] The bioethicists' arguments favor the young over the old and are designed to give everyone an opportunity to have a full life. Other things being equal, the number of years saved for a 15-year-old, for example, would far exceed the years salvaged for someone aged 75.

- Does a policy of prioritizing the young over the old for very expensive medical interventions unfairly discriminate against the elderly?

- Would it change your views if one of your parents or grandparents needed a new heart? Suppose it were your college roommate, or your child? Would it matter if the elderly person was mildly senile, or the 15-year-old was a math and science prodigy?
- Would it be better if older recipients were only eligible for older organs? For example, imagine that a 75-year-old would only be eligible for an organ from an older donor and not a heart or kidney from, say, a 25-year-old.
- While an official policy of denying the elderly expensive, scarce, life-saving therapies might be impossible to enact (given that the elderly vote while children cannot), should the elderly voluntarily forego such treatments as heart transplants out of civic duty or personal virtue to assist the next generation to achieve a full lifespan?

10. Arming Schoolteachers

Since the Columbine school shootings in Littleton, Colorado, in 1999, hundreds of people, mostly students, have been killed at different school shooting incidents. In response to this continuing tragedy, some have advocated for arming teachers as the most effective means of prevention. Others think that arming teachers creates even more hazards and that better alternatives can be found, such as more thorough background checks, curbing unregulated gun sales, and increasing mental health care for students.

- What measures for prevention of gun violence in schools do you think are morally best? Is this an issue best resolved on a school-by-school basis or through a state or national policy?
- Would the learning environment be compromised or enhanced by the knowledge that one's teacher may be carrying a gun or has a gun locked in his or her desk drawer?

- Would relationships between teachers and their students be different when teachers are armed? For example, would students be less willing to ask difficult or challenging questions of teachers or be less willing to report an incompetent teacher?

11. Paying Student-Athletes

While student-athletes routinely receive tuition scholarships, the National Collegiate Athletic Association (NCAA) has forbidden any payment to athletes that would jeopardize its aim of preserving "amateurism" in college athletics. Early in 2019 a federal judge ruled that athletes could receive more compensation, so long as it is related to education. Presumably this ruling could result in more generous stipends for books, fees, and living expenses, among other things. This ruling may also be the first step in changing the status of athletes from amateurs to professionals at elite football schools, such as Alabama, Oklahoma, and Ohio State, and elite basketball schools, such as Duke, Kentucky, and University of North Carolina at Chapel Hill. Some former and current athletes argue that the huge monetary rewards from ticket sales, television contracts, and shoe endorsements should be shared not only with the universities and their coaches, but with the athletes crucial to generating these revenues.

- Should student-athletes be considered laborers for the universities they represent, so that paying them is essentially a matter of fairness?
- Would being paid jeopardize the educational opportunities for these student-athletes?
- Only a small fraction of student-athletes, even at schools with big-revenue athletic programs, ever land a lucrative professional contract in the NBA or NFL. Should this influence our thinking pro or con about paying student-athletes?

- If paying college athletes becomes the norm, can you imagine a fair revenue-sharing formula for the student-athletes?

12. Divisive Monuments

The southeastern United States contains more than 700 memorials and statues of Confederate soldiers and wartime leaders such as Robert E. Lee, Nathan Bedford Forrest, Thomas "Stonewall" Jackson, and Jefferson Davis. These can be found in universities and public parks, within state capitol buildings, and in county courthouse squares. The Mississippi state flag still includes the Confederate battle flag in the upper left quadrant; the enormous carvings on Stone Mountain, Georgia—owned by the state—depict Lee, Jackson, and Davis on horseback. Should these statues, busts, and other monuments that celebrate or commemorate the Confederacy be removed from official buildings, public parks, and university campuses? There is a growing movement to do just that, especially from students and from African American citizens who find such statues and commemorative displays deeply offensive and symbolic of a belief in white supremacy. Some who support retaining these statues and other symbols contend that history should not be erased, and it would be wrong to remove symbols of southern historical identity.

- Should Confederate statues, busts, and commemorative plaques be removed from prominent public places or retained as reminders of the past?
- If such statues are removed from prominent public places, should they be dismantled, placed in museums as part of historical collections, or moved to graveyards as commemorative gestures to the dead? Or would some other disposition be more appropriate?

Notes

Chapter 1

1. "Two things fill the mind with ever new and increasing admiration and awe, the more often and steadily we reflect upon them: the starry heavens above me and the moral law within me." This dictum was also selected for his tombstone. Kant, *Critique of Practical Reason*, 261.
2. Hume, *Enquiry concerning the Principles of Morals*, and Smith, *Theory of Moral Sentiments*.
3. Waal, *Peacemaking Among Primates*, 270. Another insightful scholar of primate behavior is Sarah Hrdy. Her research is worth a careful look in terms of how traits of caring, helping others, sharing resources, and cooperative interdependence developed among female primates and achieved evolutionary adaptiveness among human females. See, for example, her book *Mother Nature*.
4. The basis of Socrates' wisdom is the recognition of his ignorance amid the many false claims to knowledge by the "experts" around him. See *Apology*, 23a, trans. Hugh Tredenick, in Plato, *Collected Dialogues*, 9.
5. "All things are in motion and nothing at rest, [like the stream of a river] you cannot go into the same water twice" is how Plato talks of Heraclitus's teaching. See *Cratylus*, 402a, trans. Benjamin Jowett, in Plato, *Collected Dialogues*, 439.
6. Blackburn, *Being Good*, 19–29.
7. Blackburn, *Being Good*, 48–49.
8. Montaigne, *Complete Essays*, 856.
9. Nagel, *Equality and Partiality*, 6.
10. Descartes, *Rules for the Direction of the Mind*.

Chapter 2

1. Most moral development schemes are heavily shaped by moral theory. Those of Piaget and Kohlberg are perhaps the most obvious examples, as both are explicitly indebted to Kant and to changes in reasoning processes

as the important developmental thresholds. In speaking of a "prehistory" and the effort to interrogate it, I would like to avoid or minimize theoretical sponsorship and simply describe, with few assumptions, a phenomenon I think most people would readily recognize as a feature of moving from childhood and adolescence into adulthood. An additional reason for minimizing theory in models for moral development is that they often become expressions of romanticized understandings of the moral self, moving from ignorance or error to moral enlightenment in a highly truncated process. For example, think here of the vanity involved (and the moral hazards!) in moral accounts that assume we are always the protagonists, or better, the heroes, in an imagined life progression, involving some pivotal insight about the true nature of the Right or the Good. We might call this the "road to Damascus" model for moral development. Religious narratives of moral selfhood may be especially prone to this, but one need not be religious to fall prey to this sort of self-congratulatory story.
2. I am not referring here to "prehistory" in the way that archeologists or evolutionary biologists might think of the prehistory of the human species, meaning the time before humans began to keep written records. "Prehistory" as I use it here is a way of referencing the defining moral influences that shaped each of us, individually, before we were aware of being shaped. Thus, it is not so much prewriting as it is prereflective.
3. Among many of Berry's writings that emphasize the moral importance of place, see his collection of essays *What Are People For?*
4. See Basso, *Wisdom Sits in Places*, esp. chap. 4.
5. Among the important works in ethics that stress the social sense of self are Niebuhr, *Responsible Self*; Buber, *I and Thou*; and the major ethical works of the Scottish Enlightenment, viz., Hume, *Enquiry Concerning the Principles of Morals*, and Smith, *Theory of Moral Sentiments*.
6. David Brooks, "The Moral Bucket List," New York Times, April 11, 2015.
7. Two important books address the power and influence of pharmaceutical and device companies on physician practices, the conflicts of interest they create in physicians and the moral maneuvering many physicians use to try to justify the acceptance of what are essentially bribes and kickbacks. See Kassirer, *On the Take*, and Angell, *Truth About the Drug Companies*.
8. See AMA Council on Ethical and Judicial Affairs, "AMA Code of Medical Ethics' Opinions."
9. See Grande et al., "Effect of Exposure to Small Pharmaceutical Promotional Items on Treatment Preferences."

10. Shepherd, "The Hair Stylist, the Corn Merchant, and the Doctor."
11. Halperin, Hutchison, and Barrier, "Population-Based Study of the Prevalence and Influence of Gifts to Radiation Oncologists from Pharmaceutical Companies and Medical Equipment Manufacturers." In this study, only 5 percent of physicians thought their own prescribing habits were affected by receiving gifts, but 33 percent thought the practices of their colleagues were affected.
12. Blackburn, *Mirror, Mirror*, 189. This entire book will repay a careful reading.
13. Empathy is increasingly the subject of social scientific study. For example, Simon Baron-Cohen argues in his book *Zero Degrees of Empathy* that the concept of evil should be replaced by "empathy erosion." Baron-Cohen's argument is finally too reductionist to be fully convincing, yet his studies do help us understand more fully the importance of empathy in moral behavior.
14. Whitman, *Democratic Vistas*, 337.
15. Mill, *Utilitarianism*, 376ff.
16. Kant, *Foundations of the Metaphysics of Morals*, 22–59.
17. Von Blum, *Civil Rights for Beginners*, 14–45.
18. Pascal, *Pensées*, 16. Pascal was writing about the fluctuating nature of human thinking based on locale, but also on seasonal and astrological changes, so his point is more commodious to my emphasis on personal temporal flux than it might at first appear.
19. Merleau-Ponty, *Phenomenology of Perception*, 346.
20. This is a point made in greater detail in Churchill and Simán, "Principles and the Search for Moral Certainty."
21. Phaedrus, 246b, trans. R. Hackforth, in Plato, *Collected Dialogues*, 483ff.
22. Kant, *Foundations of the Metaphysics of Morals*, 3–14.
23. See Luke 10:33–35, in May and Metzger, *Oxford Annotated Bible*, 1259ff.
24. Kass, "Wisdom of Repugnance."
25. Kahneman, *Thinking, Fast and Slow*.
26. Kahneman, *Thinking, Fast and Slow*, 13–14.

Chapter 3

1. Sobel, "Beyond Empathy," 471.
2. Waal, *The Bonobo and the Atheist*, 52, 82.
3. Sobel, "Beyond Empathy," 474–76.

4. I do not argue that the Enlightenment in America was without major moral flaws and even systematic cruelties. Jefferson, for example, was in many ways a product of his time and shared in its tyrannies. He held slaves and treated women with far less than full moral regard. Enlightenment periods typically cast a long shadow in which moral evil persists, and Jefferson's iconic status serves as a reminder of both noble aspirations and residual crimes.
5. Kant, "What Is Enlightenment?"
6. Hobbes, *Of Man*.
7. Kant, *Foundations of the Metaphysics of Morals*, 9ff.
8. See https://link.springer.com/journal/10902.
9. See https://www.happinessresearchinstitute.com/.
10. Aristotle, *Nicomachean Ethics*, 1115a6–1117a28, in McKeon, *Basic Works of Aristotle*, 974–79.
11. For excellent accounts of the importance of narrative and storytelling in ethics, see Charon and Montello, *Stories Matter*; Brody, *Stories of Sickness*; and Charon, *Narrative Medicine*.

Chapter 4

1. I wrote an earlier version of these prompts for inclusion in admission interviews at Vanderbilt University Medical School a decade ago. I thank Drs. John Zic and Bonnie Miller for their encouragement in devising such prompts and for their conviction that some effort to measure moral sensitivity and development is important.

Chapter 5

1. Freedman, "Offering Truth."
2. Kant, *Foundations of the Metaphysics of Morals*, 17.
3. Epictetus, *Art of Living*. Editor Sharon Lebell's interpretation reads: "Happiness and freedom begin with a clear understanding of one principle: Some things are within our control, and some things are not" (p. 3). Most things are not. Yet "we always have a choice about the contents and character of our inner lives" (p. 3). And an admonition: "Trying to control or to change what we can't only results in torment" (p. 3).
4. Gilligan, *In a Different Voice*.
5. Taylor, *Philosophy and the Human Sciences*, 244.
6. Pfaff, *Neuroscience of Fair Play*, 61ff.

7. See Butler, "Sermon II, III—Upon the Natural Supremacy of Conscience."
8. Marcel, *Mystery of Being*.
9. Porter, "Marriage Is Belonging," 792–93.

Chapter 6

1. Bok, *Lying*, 22.
2. Bok, *Lying*, 25.
3. See https://en.oxforddictionaries.com/definition/post-truth (accessed on August 20, 2018).
4. Dickens, *Great Expectations*.
5. Arendt, *Human Condition*, 238.
6. Arendt, *Human Condition*, 240.
7. Arendt, *Human Condition*, 241.
8. Wiesenthal, *Sunflower*.
9. Nussbaum, *Love's Knowledge*, 336–37.
10. Ruddick, *Maternal Thinking*.
11. Held, *Ethics of Care*.
12. Kittay, *Love's Labor*.
13. Whitman, *Leaves of Grass*, 36.
14. Otto, *Idea of the Holy*.
15. Eliade, *Cosmos and History*.
16. Wach, *Comparative Study of Religions*.
17. James, *Varieties of Religious Experience*.
18. Maslow, *Religions, Values, and Peak-Experiences*.
19. Whitman, *Leaves of Grass*, 76.
20. Aristotle, *Nicomachean Ethics* 3.7, 1116a2–1116a6, in McKeon, *Basic Works of Aristotle*, 976.
21. Andre, *Worldly Virtues*, 41.
22. Eagleton, *Hope without Optimism*, 1–38.
23. Andre, *Worldly Virtues*, 40.
24. Marcel, *Homo Viator*, 29–67.
25. Lear, *Radical Hope*.
26. Andre, *Worldly Virtues*, 31–44.

Chapter 7

1. Fingarette, *On Responsibility*, 42.
2. Feuerbach, *Essence of Christianity*, 12–32.

3. Firth, "Ethical Absolutism and the Ideal Observer."
4. Smith, *Theory of Moral Sentiments*, 83.
5. Hobbes, *Of Man*, 405.
6. Rawls, *Theory of Justice*, 302–3.
7. Henry, "Liberty or Death."
8. Berlin, *Two Concepts of Liberty*.
9. Mill, *On Liberty*, 9.
10. King, "Glossary of Basic Ethical Concepts in Health Care and Research," 161.
11. Kant, *Foundations of the Metaphysics of Morals*, 53.
12. Singer, *Animal Liberation*.
13. Regan, *Case for Animal Rights*.
14. Dworkin, *Taking Rights Seriously*.
15. Bennett, "Conscience of Huckleberry Finn."
16. Dickinson, *Poems*, 682.
17. Stevens, "Sunday Morning," 69.
18. Homer, *Odyssey*, 93–94.
19. For an insightful interpretation of Odysseus's choice, see John Churchill, "Odysseus's Bed." "Odysseus's leaving Calypso signifies a loyalty to humanity—to the inexorable patterns of birth, reproduction, and death in whose context alone we can recognize a life that we could claim as our own" (p. 7).
20. Nussbaum, *Fragility of Goodness*, 2, interpreting Pindar's *Nemean*.
21. Seneca, "Letter 26."
22. Montaigne, *Complete Essays*, 64.

Chapter 8

1. Coral Davenport, "Major Climate Report Describes a Strong Risk of Crisis as Early as 2040," *New York Times,* October 7, 2018.
2. Coral Davenport and Kendra Pierre-Louis, "U.S. Climate Report Warns of Damaged Environment and Shrinking Economy," *New York Times*, November 23, 2018.
3. Gardiner, *Perfect Moral Storm*, 123. See also Hardin, "Tragedy of the Commons." Hardin asks us to imagine a common pasture that is open to free grazing. Each herdsman calculates that it is in his best interest to keep as many cattle on the commons as possible, since gains to him from selling the cattle are all his, but the cost of feeding them is shared by all the herdsmen. Each herdsman follows this logic and increases his herd. The commons, however vast it may seem initially, is limited. Eventually,

each herdsman pursuing his individual best interest leads inexorably to depleted grazing where few can survive. Gardiner thinks the global warming problem is an even worse version of such a tragedy because it develops over multiple generations and is thereby more hidden in a single lifespan.
4. Gardiner, *Perfect Moral Storm*, 143.
5. Jennings, *Ecological Governance*, 166–67.
6. David Leonhardt, "The Problem with Putting a Price on the End of the World," *New York Times Magazine*, April 9, 2019.
7. Jamieson, *Reason in a Dark Time*, 237.
8. Brown, *Climate Change Ethics*, 226.
9. Saffo, "Accidental Elegance."
10. Mill, *On Liberty*.
11. Berger, *Ways of Seeing*. For an extensive description of the many areas of life invaded by consumerism and commercial values, see Sandel, *What Money Can't Buy*.
12. McDaniel, *Living from the Center*, 13.
13. McDaniel, *Living from the Center*, 15.
14. Durning, *How Much Is Enough?* 149.
15. Nagel, *View from Nowhere*.
16. Benhabib, "The Generalized and the Concrete Other," 163–71.
17. Merleau-Ponty, "Unpublished Text," 3.
18. See, for example, I Corinthians 7, which also lends support for the church's long-standing misogyny.
19. Plato's teachings on the soul/body dichotomy are most clearly expressed in *Phaedrus*, *Phaedo*, and *The Republic*.
20. This quote from Gould is taken from Orr, *Earth in Mind*, 43. Orr's book also devotes a short chapter to love, in which he discusses Wilson's notion of biophilia, arguing that this urge to affiliate with other life forms must become a conscious part of what we think and do environmentally. See "Love," in Orr, *Earth in Mind*, 43–47. I think this is a move in the right direction, but falls short of what is needed. See note 23.
21. Heschel, *Essential Writings*, 51.
22. Niebuhr, *Responsible Self*, 118–19.
23. A kindred notion has been discussed in evolutionary terms by Edward O. Wilson in his book *Biophilia*, although "biophilia" is usually understood as an urge to affiliate with other life forms. As an urge it may not be self-conscious, and it also may not involve the deep affective dimension I believe is needed to spur environmental action.

24. Sacks, *Gratitude*, 20.
25. Callenbach, "Earth's 10 Commandments."
26. Grinspoon, *Earth in Human Hands*, 77. The whole of chapter 2 in Grinspoon's book, "Can a Planet Be Alive?" should be required reading for all serious people.

Chapter 9

1. The Terri Schiavo case is a right-to-die case that played out in the United States between 1990 and 2005 and concerned a woman who suffered heart failure, was rescued, but subsequently remained in a permanent vegetative state (PVS). Ms. Schiavo's husband and legal guardian worked assiduously for her rehabilitation, but he also argued that she would not want to be sustained on prolonged artificial life support and took action to remove her feeding tube. Ms. Schiavo had left no advance care planning documents. Her parents disagreed about both the diagnosis of PVS and what her wishes would be regarding artificial life support. The ensuing legal battles captured international media attention, as well as efforts of then U.S. president George W. Bush and legislative efforts by Jeb Bush, then governor of Florida, to keep Ms. Schiavo's feeding tube in place. Following a lengthy legal review, Terri Schiavo's feeding tube was removed, and she died on March 31, 2005. The postmortem examination confirmed the PVS diagnosis and showed that her brain had liquified.
2. The Enron Corporation case is the story of a company that reached great heights and then suffered a complete collapse because of corporate corruption. At its peak the Houston-based energy company's stock traded for over $90 a share. After its corruption was exposed the value of a share fell to $0.26. Enron was formed in 1985 by Kenneth Lay after merging Houston Natural Gas and InterNorth. Several years later, when Jeffrey Skilling was hired, he developed a staff of executives that hid billions of dollars in debt from failed deals and projects. Chief Financial Officer Andrew Fastow and other executives not only misled Enron's board of directors and audit committee with high-risk accounting practices but also pressured Enron's auditors, Arthur Andersen, to ignore the issues. Many executives at Enron were indicted on a variety of charges, and some were later sentenced to prison. Arthur Andersen was found guilty of illegally destroying documents relevant to the Security and Exchange Commission investigation. As a result, Arthur Anderson's license to audit public companies was voided, and the firm effectively closed. Enron employees and shareholders

received limited returns in lawsuits, despite losing billions in pensions and stock prices. As a consequence of the scandal, new regulations and legislation were enacted to enhance the accuracy of financial reporting for public companies.
3. The trolley problem is a famous thought experiment in ethics. The typical form it takes is as follows. There is a runaway trolley moving toward five unaware or incapacitated people on the tracks. You can pull a lever and divert the trolley to a side track. On the side track, it will kill only one person rather than five. What is the more ethical choice? There are also variations on this scenario, for example, pushing a fat man onto the track, thereby killing him but stopping the trolley. Alternatively, the case is sometimes described such that you have a close relationship to the one person on the diverted side track. Philippa Foot, an early twentieth-century Oxford philosopher, is usually credited with inventing the problem, although it has been discussed by a number of prominent contemporary philosophers. It is also a popular example for researchers doing empirical studies in moral psychology.
4. Chambers, *Fiction of Bioethics*, 177–78.
5. See, for example, Callahan, *Setting Limits*.

Bibliography

AMA Council on Ethical and Judicial Affairs. "AMA Code of Medical Ethics' Opinions on Physicians' Relationships with Drug Companies and Duty to Assist in Containing Drug Costs." *Virtual Mentor* 16 (2014): 261–64.

Andre, Judith. *Worldly Virtues: Moral Ideals and Contemporary Life.* Lanham, MD: Lexington Books, 2015.

Angell, Marcia. *The Truth about the Drug Companies: How They Deceive Us and What to Do about It.* New York: Random House, 2004.

Arendt, Hannah. *The Human Condition.* Chicago: University of Chicago Press, 1958.

Aristotle. *Nicomachean Ethics.* Translated by W. D. Ross. In *The Basic Works of Aristotle.* Edited by Richard McKeon, 935–1112. New York: Random House, 1941.

Baron-Cohen, Simon. *Zero Degrees of Empathy: A New Theory of Human Cruelty.* London: Penguin, 2011.

Basso, Keith H. *Wisdom Sits in Places: Landscape and Language among the Western Apache.* Albuquerque: University of New Mexico Press, 1996.

Benhabib, Seyla. "The Generalized and the Concrete Other: The Kohlberg-Gilligan Controversy and Moral Theory." In *Women and Moral Theory.* Edited by Eva Feder Kittay and Diana T. Meyers, 154–77. Totowa, NJ: Rowman and Littlefield, 1987.

Bennett, Jonathan. "The Conscience of Huckleberry Finn." *Philosophy* 49 (April 1974): 123–34.

Berger, John. *Ways of Seeing.* New York: Penguin, 1977.

Berlin, Isaiah. *Two Concepts of Liberty.* Oxford: Clarendon Press, 1959.

Berry, Wendell. *What Are People For?* Berkeley, CA: Counterpoint, 2010.

Blackburn, Simon. *Being Good: A Short Introduction to Ethics.* New York: Oxford University Press, 2001.

Blackburn, Simon. *Mirror, Mirror: The Uses and Abuses of Self-Love.* Princeton, NJ: Princeton University Press, 2014.

Bok, Sissela. *Lying: Moral Choice in Public and Private Life.* New York: Pantheon Books, 1978.

Brody, Howard. *Stories of Sickness.* 2nd ed. New York: Oxford University Press, 2002.

Brown, Donald A. *Climate Change Ethics: Navigating the Perfect Moral Storm.* New York: Routledge, 2013.

Buber, Martin. *I and Thou*. Translated by Walter Kaufmann. New York: Charles Scribner's Sons, 1970.
Butler, Joseph. "Sermon II, III—Upon the Natural Supremacy of Conscience." In *British Moralists, 1650–1800*. Vol. 1. Edited by D. D. Raphael, 346–61. Oxford: Oxford University Press, 1969.
Callahan, Daniel. *Setting Limits: Medical Goals in an Aging Society*. New York: Simon and Schuster, 1987.
Callenbach, Ernest. "Earth's 10 Commandments." In *The Poster Art of David Lance Goines: A 40-Year Retrospective*. By Ernest Callenbach, 80. Mineola, NY: Dover, 2010.
Chambers, Tod. *The Fiction of Bioethics: Cases as Literary Texts*. New York: Routledge, 1999.
Charon, Rita. *Narrative Medicine: Honoring the Stories of Illness*. New York: Oxford University Press, 2006.
Charon, Rita, and Martha Montello, eds. *Stories Matter: The Role of Narrative in Medical Ethics*. New York: Routledge, 2002.
Churchill, John. "Odysseus's Bed; Agamemnon's Bath." *College Literature* 18, no. 1 (1991): 1–13.
Churchill, Larry R., and José Jorge Simán. "Principles and the Search for Moral Certainty." *Social Science and Medicine* 23, no. 5 (1986): 461–68.
Descartes, René. *Rules for the Direction of the Mind*. In *The Philosophical Works of Descartes*. Vol. 1. Translated by Elizabeth S Haldane and G. R. T. Ross, 1–77. Cambridge, UK: Cambridge University Press, 1970.
Dickens, Charles. *Great Expectations*. Edited by Charlotte Mitchell. London: Penguin Classics, 1996.
Dickinson, Emily. *Emily Dickinson's Poems: As She Preserved Them*. Edited by Cristanne Miller. Cambridge, MA: Belknap Press of Harvard University Press, 2016.
Durning, Alan. *How Much Is Enough? The Consumer Society and the Future of the Earth*. New York: Norton, 1992.
Dworkin, Ronald. *Taking Rights Seriously*. Cambridge, MA: Harvard University Press, 1977.
Eagleton, Terry *Hope without Optimism*. Charlottesville: University of Virginia Press, 2015.
Eliade, Mircea. *Cosmos and History: The Myth of the Eternal Return*. Translated by Willard Trask. New York: Harper and Brothers, 1954.
Epictetus. *The Art of Living: The Classic Manual on Virtue, Happiness, and Effectiveness*. Edited by Sharon Lebell. San Francisco, CA: HarperSanFrancisco, 1995.
Feuerbach, Ludwig. *The Essence of Christianity*. Translated by George Eliot. New York: Harper and Brothers, 1957.
Fingarette, Herbert. *On Responsibility*. New York: Basic Books, 1967.

Firth, Roderick. "Ethical Absolutism and the Ideal Observer." *Philosophy and Phenomenological Research* 12, no. 3 (1952): 317–45.
Freedman, Benjamin. "Offering Truth: One Ethical Approach to the Uninformed Cancer Patient." *Archives of Internal Medicine* 153, no. 5 (1993): 572–76.
Gardiner, Stephen M. *A Perfect Moral Storm: The Ethical Tragedy of Climate Change.* New York: Oxford University Press, 2011.
Gilligan. Carol. *In a Different Voice: Psychological Theory and Women's Development.* Cambridge, MA: Harvard University Press, 1982.
Grande, David, Dominick L. Frosch, Andrew W. Perkins, and Barbara E. Kahn. "Effect of Exposure to Small Pharmaceutical Promotional Items on Treatment Preferences." *Archives of Internal Medicine* 169, no. 9 (2009): 887–93.
Grinspoon, David. *Earth in Human Hands: Shaping Our Planet's Future.* New York: Grand Central, 2016.
Halperin, Edward C., Paul Hutchison, and Robert C. Barrier Jr. "A Population-Based Study of the Prevalence and Influence of Gifts to Radiation Oncologists from Pharmaceutical Companies and Medical Equipment Manufacturers." *International Journal of Radiation Oncology, Biology, Physics* 59, no. 5 (2004): 1477–83.
Hardin, Garrett. "The Tragedy of the Commons." *Science* 162, no. 3859 (1968): 1243–248.
Held, Virginia. *The Ethics of Care: Personal, Political, and Global.* New York: Oxford University Press, 2006.
Henry, Patrick. "Liberty or Death." In *Great American Speeches.* Edited by Gregory R. Suriano, 1–4. New York: Gramercy Books, 1993.
Heschel, Abraham Joshua. *Abraham Joshua Heschel: Essential Writings.* Edited by Susannah Heschel. Maryknoll, NY: Orbis Books, 2011.
Hobbes, Thomas. *Of Man, Being the First Part of Leviathan.* In *French and English Philosophers: Descartes, Rousseau, Voltaire, Hobbs.* Edited by Charles W. Eliot, 323–434. New York: P. F. Collier, 1910.
Homer. *The Odyssey of Homer.* Translated by Richard Lattimore. New York: Harper and Row, 1965.
Hrdy, Sarah Blaffer. *Mother Nature: Maternal Instincts and How They Shape the Human Species.* New York: Ballantine, 2000.
Hume, David. *An Enquiry concerning the Principles of Morals.* 2nd ed. La Salle, IL: Open Court, 1966.
James, William. *The Varieties of Religious Experience.* Marston Gate, UK: Renaissance Classics, 2012.
Jamieson, Dale. *Reason in a Dark Time: Why the Struggle against Climate Change Failed—and What It Means for Our Future.* New York: Oxford University Press, 2014.
Jennings, Bruce. *Ecological Governance: Toward a New Social Contract with the Earth.* Morgantown: West Virginia University Press, 2016.

Kahneman, Daniel. *Thinking, Fast and Slow*. New York: Farrar, Straus and Giroux, 2011.
Kant, Immanuel. *Critique of Practical Reason*. In *The Philosophy of Kant: Immanuel Kant's Moral and Political Writings*. Translated by Carl J. Friedrich, 209–64. New York: Modern Library, 1949.
Kant, Immanuel. *Foundations of the Metaphysics of Morals*. Translated by Lewis White Beck. New York: Macmillan, 1985.
Kant, Immanuel. "What Is Enlightenment?" In *Foundations of the Metaphysics of Morals*. By Emmanuel Kant. Translated by Lewis White Beck, 85–92. New York: Macmillan, 1985.
Kass, Leon R. "The Wisdom of Repugnance: Why We Should Ban the Cloning of Humans." *New Republic* 216, no. 22 (1997): 17–26.
Kassirer, Jerome P. *On the Take: How Medicine's Complicity with Big Business Can Endanger Your Health*. New York: Oxford University Press, 2005.
King, Nancy M. P. "Glossary of Basic Ethical Concepts in Health Care and Research." In *The Social Medicine Reader*. Vol. 1, *Patients, Doctors, and Illness*. 2nd ed. Edited by Nancy M. P. King, Ronald P. Strauss, Larry R. Churchill, Sue E. Estroff, Gail E. Henderson, and Jonathan Oberlander, 161–68. Durham, NC: Duke University Press, 2005.
Kittay, Eva Feder. *Love's Labor: Essays on Women, Equality, and Dependency*. New York: Routledge, 1999.
Lear, Jonathan. *Radical Hope: Ethics in the Face of Cultural Devastation*. Cambridge, MA: Harvard University Press, 2006.
Marcel, Gabriel. *Homo Viator: Introduction to a Metaphysic of Hope*. Translated by Emma Craufurd. Gloucester, MA: Peter Smith, 1978.
Marcel, Gabriel. *The Mystery of Being*. Vol. 1, *Reflection and Mystery*. Translated by G. S. Fraser. London: Harvill Press, 1950.
Maslow, Abraham H. *Religions, Values, and Peak-Experiences*. Columbus: Ohio State University Press, 1964.
May, Herbert G., and Bruce M Metzger, eds. *The Oxford Annotated Bible, with the Apocrypha*. Rev. Standard Version. New York: Oxford University Press, 1965.
McDaniel, Jay. *Living from the Center: Spirituality in an Age of Consumerism*. St. Louis, MO: Chalice Press, 2000.
Merleau-Ponty, Maurice. *Phenomenology of Perception*. Translated by Colin Smith. London: Routledge and Kegan Paul, 1962.
Merleau-Ponty, Maurice. "An Unpublished Text by Maurice Merleau-Ponty: A Prospectus of His Work." Translated by Arleen B. Dallery. In *The Primacy of Perception, and Other Essays on Phenomenological Psychology, the Philosophy of Art, History and Politics*. Edited by James M. Edie, 3–11. Evanston, IL: Northwestern University Press, 1964.
Mill, John Stuart. *On Liberty*. Edited by Elizabeth Rapaport. Indianapolis, IN: Hackett, 1978.